D1637684

The Dark Side

Real Life Accounts of an NHS Paramedic
The Good, the Bad and the Downright Ugly

Andy Thompson

****

Also Available

The Dark Side Part 2
Real Life Accounts of an NHS Paramedic
The Traumatic, the Tragic and the Tearful

Published in September 2014 by emp3books,
Norwood House, Elvetham Road, Fleet, GU51 4HL, England

The Dark Side

Real Life Accounts of an NHS Paramedic
The Good, the Bad and the Downright Ugly
by Andy Thompson

Digital edition first published in 2013 by The Electronic Book Company

ISBN: 978-1-907140-33-4

Dedication

This book is dedicated to my beautiful wife Emma, for her support and encouragement throughout its production; and to all those Health Care Professionals around the globe who, where possible, save life and work tirelessly to help make a difference to their sick and injured patients.

About the Author

In June 2002, Andy commenced employment with the Mersey Regional Ambulance Service, which later merged with the Cumbria, Greater Manchester and Lancashire Ambulance Services to form the Northwest Ambulance Service NHS Trust. He rapidly progressed from the Patient Transport Service (PTS) to qualified Paramedic status via Ambulance Technician training, experience gained in the job and further extended training from which, upon qualifying, he was presented with a 'Professional Paramedic Development Award' for most improved candidate.

In 2005 he registered with the Health Professions Council (HPC), the national governing body for UK paramedics; this changed its name to the Health and Care Professions Council (HCPC) in August 2012.

Andy spent the earlier part of his career working in the English counties of Cheshire and Merseyside. In 2007, after living 'up north' for 32 years, Andy relocated down south with his wife and two children, residing there until he and his family relocated to North Yorkshire in September 2013. There, Andy continues his career as an NHS Paramedic with the Yorkshire Ambulance Service.

To read more about the author, please visit:
www.andythompson-author.com

Contents

Dedication iii

About the Author iv

Prologue... vii

Introduction 1

Chapter 1   Baptism of Fire.................... 3

Chapter 2   A Thousand Mile Journey 23

Chapter 3   Hindsight.......................... 41

Chapter 4   Shutdown 59

Chapter 5   Left for Dead 79

Chapter 6   A Fateful Decision............... 97

Chapter 7   An Undignified Death............. 109

Chapter 8   Something's Not Right!........... 119

Chapter 9   As Thick as Thieves............. 133

Chapter 10   Sweet Dreams 151

Epilogue.. 161

Layman's Terms.................................... 163

The Dark Side

Prologue

The incidents I have written about in this book are a selection of real life accounts of situations I have experienced during my career in the NHS Ambulance Service, and what is written is as true and honest as my long-term memory will serve me, supported by the *precise* details taken from anonymised copies of the official NHS documentation I recorded at the time of each incident. Furthermore, the dialogue quoted in each chapter is also true to what remains in my long-term memory; however, I do not profess it to be verbatim.

The Dark Side

Introduction

'The Dark Side' – an unofficial term used by Mersey Regional Ambulance Service personnel to describe the career transition from the non-emergency aspect, to the frontline emergency aspect, of the Ambulance Service; pertaining to the fact that what one frequently encounters is often a grim and sombre experience.

'I couldn't do your job. I bet you've seen allsorts, haven't you?'

If I was given a penny for every time someone has said that to me, I'd have... er... erm... one pound eighty-seven pence by now. I jest. I can't honestly say how many times that has been said to me, but I hear it that often that I usually reply with 'I know you couldn't, you're not qualified.' In all seriousness though, there is no doubt that being a paramedic would certainly not suit everybody. Of course, not everybody would want to be a paramedic; that goes without saying.

That's not to say people don't take an interest in the work of paramedics and what they encounter on a daily basis. Over the last ten years or so, there have been numerous fly-on-the-wall documentaries on television following the day-to-day working lives of ambulance personnel, and a variety of blog-based books released too; so there is obviously some demand or none of them would have been produced. Though, unfortunately, the documentaries seldom depict a true picture of what the job is really like. The true-to-life material is usually found on the cutting room floor, classed as too inappropriate for television. The books, however, paint a more accurate picture about what it's like to be a paramedic, but none of them tend to go in to detail about the patient encounter.

With all that in mind, I decided to pen a selection of my own personal memoirs, from the experiences that have remained with me through no choice of my own; they've become engraved, for

1

one reason only – because they are all unforgettable.

As already mentioned, I have used anonymised copies of the official NHS documentation I recorded at the time of each incident to include *precise* details. I sometimes retained anonymised copies of particularly interesting incidents because, as a Registered Health Care Professional, I have to maintain my fitness to practice, and so I possess a Continuous Professional Development (CPD) portfolio containing a wide variety of work-based evidence and reflective practice essays. The Health and Care Professions Council (HCPC) undertake a random audit on its registrants every two years, and require submitted evidence to be within the last two years of clinical practice from the date of audit.

However, since qualifying as a paramedic in 2005, my name has not yet been pulled out of the hat, so to speak. Needless to say, the photocopies that I have – the same ones I had intended to write a reflective piece on for my CPD portfolio – are now obsolete, for audit purposes that is, but not for allowing me to include specific details while writing my paramedical memoirs. I suppose this book could become the most in-depth, detailed and descriptive piece of reflective work I'll ever own; and will inevitably replace the creased, scrap photocopies I have hoarded in a Lever Arch File in the loft for several years.

There are no heroics in this book; I simply did my job and what is expected of me during each shift. I did what *most* paramedics around the globe would do, and I'm sure *most* paramedics will relate to the incidents I've written about.

So, while I go and get ready for another unpredictable twelve hour shift, go and grab yourself a cuppa, sit back and put your feet up, and imagine you're on duty with me, donning a fluorescent jacket with the title 'Observer' emblazoned across the back. It might just change your perspective on life, and add a harsh reminder of why you should live life to the full, and live every day as if it was your last.

Chapter 1
Baptism of Fire

Just a short time had gone by since I'd finished my paramedic training course, and I was still wet behind the ears, soaking in fact – in terms of paramedic experience, that is. I'd had very little cause to use my new found skills thus far. As an ambulance technician (a paramedic's assistant) I'd experienced the same things as my paramedic peers, granted, but most of the time I had a paramedic to turn to when the shit hit the fan. *I* was now the one that the technician would turn to when the shit hit the fan.

It didn't seem that long ago since I was walking the streets, and donkey's years away from becoming a paramedic. Where had the time gone? It had flown by, that's where, and I'd achieved my ambition, with health care professional registration and paramedic epaulettes to prove it. The responsibility of being the most qualified and skilled member of an ambulance crew, where my clinical decisions could make the difference between life and death, was daunting to say the least, but nonetheless about to begin. And unfortunately for me, the sheer reality of the responsibility I had came in the form of trauma – my *Baptism of Fire*. Allow me to share that experience with you, in considerable detail.

I was approaching the end of a twelve hour night shift on overtime. My crewmate, Adam, a very good friend of mine, was still a rookie; he'd not long transferred to The Dark Side and was still learning his trade as a probationary ambulance technician. Adam was a great character with a fantastic sense of humour, and also an eye for the ladies!

We had not stopped all night, nor had any of the other crews from the same station. We had all been responding to treble-nine after treble-nine, and were absolutely exhausted. We were all sat together in the station mess room chatting and drinking tea. It was

6:45a.m. and we all eagerly awaited our relief staff, who historically would arrive fifteen minutes before the start of their shift. But they had not, so me and Adam were sitting ducks to cop a late treble-nine, as we were the next crew out if an emergency call came in. Another five minutes passed by and there was still no sign of our relief crew. Then, to my disappointment, my hand portable radio sounded.

'Oh, bloody 'ell!' I said, before pressing the push-to-talk button, 'Receiving, over.'

'Roger, RED call to a single vehicle RTC near the junction of Gaspar Lane. One patient reported; police on route too, over,' the dispatcher said.

'Roger that,' I replied.

Adam and I had no choice but to respond immediately. Now the next crew out were on tenterhooks, as their relief crew had not arrived either. So me and Adam exited the station and adopted our appointed positions in the ambulance – him driving and me in the attendant's seat. As we moved off with blue lights flashing, our relief crew were just getting out of their cars. Adam looked at me with a cunning expression.

'Forget it mate, we'll have to go now,' I said, with temptation to do what Adam was thinking and ask the crew to respond to the RTC for us. I don't know what it was, but I had a sixth sense and thought to myself that it was probably best that we go, as the relief crew were a double technician crew and the incident location had a sixty mile per hour speed limit. This could be very serious and require paramedic intervention.

We drove the three miles to the crash scene, with the blue lights flashing and sirens wailing, chatting along the way but dazed.

'It'll probably be some daft sod with a dent in his car, rubbing his 'ed,' Adam remarked.

'We'll see mate, we'll see,' I replied, less hopeful and an anticipatory sixth sense still lingering. When we rolled up to the scene, a bystander approached the ambulance, so I wound down the window.

'Where's the crash, mate?' I asked.

'Over there,' the bystander said, pointing at a large field.

'Are the police on scene?'

'Yeah, there's a copper with him.'

'OK, cheers mate.'

So me and Adam got out of the ambulance, opened up the side door and grabbed the oxygen and the paramedic bag. While doing that we could see a male lying flat on his back, about twenty-five yards across the field, and a copper kneeling next to him, immobilising his head. But we couldn't see any scene of a collision anywhere, which confused us both. We casually walked towards the patient and the copper, carrying our equipment. From a distance it wasn't clear whether the patient had any injuries or not. As we progressed along the field, we spotted the patient's Subaru to our left; it was a mangled heap of carnage, crunched against a tree.

'It's gonna be a youngster,' I said to Adam, before pausing momentarily. 'Hang on… why isn't he still in the car?' I curiously asked, thinking out aloud but knowing full well Adam would be as clueless as I was. With damage like that, I thought, the occupant should either be dead, trapped or at the very least still inside. It looked like the car had smashed through a fence and come to a sudden halt with the assistance of a tree that must have been hundreds of years old, judging by the size of the trunk. As we got nearer to the patient, an audible sucking sound resonated through my ears. That doesn't sound good, I thought.

'Ohhh shhhit,' I said to Adam with my teeth clenched together in a ventriloquist-like manner. My heart rate more than doubled, from a normal sixty beats per minute (60bpm) to about one hundred and fifty (150bpm) within seconds. I could feel it thumping against my chest, as if trying to escape from inside me, and my lungs suddenly demanded more oxygen. Adrenaline was the cause.

I understood adrenaline. Having a broad interest in self-defence and the fighting arts for many years, I'd studied it in some detail, particularly the side effects of it, and also how to control it. But that's the hardest part; it's difficult to control the side effects. If adrenaline is not understood and controlled, it can cause you to freeze on the spot, and panic will set in. The more you panic, the greater the adrenaline release. The greater the adrenaline release, the more you panic. The only way to control adrenaline is to accept its purpose, accept it's there to help you to get through a stressful situation.

You see, adrenaline is a hormone produced by the adrenal glands during high stress or exciting situations. This powerful hormone is part of the human body's acute stress response system, also called the 'fight or flight' response. It works by stimulating the heart rate, contracting blood vessels, and dilating air passages, all of which work to increase blood flow to the muscles and oxygen to the lungs. However, adrenaline is often mistaken for fear, not only by the person experiencing the adrenal release, but also by those watching. For instance, during a confrontation or a verbal or physical attack, exposing the effects of adrenaline to your potential attacker is often perceived by *you*, and them, as *you* being scared or weak. But it's as natural as blinking and nothing to be ashamed of or embarrassed about. The assailant will be feeling the same effects too but attempts to hide them with aggressive verbal and mobile body language, such as splaying the arms out to the sides and pacing about to appear bigger and more threatening, thus hiding *his* trembling hands and legs.

Our Neanderthal ancestors would have felt the side effects of adrenaline too, but they would have faced a killer beast, with the odds stacked heavily against them if they didn't run. Now, in the twenty-first century, our bodies consider something as non-life-threatening as a driving test as a threat to one's life. So our adrenal glands secrete adrenaline to assist us, to give us the option to either take the driving test (fight), or tell the examiner to shove it up his arse, and then take the bus home instead (flight).

Unfortunately, the side effects of adrenaline do not help under the circumstances often faced by a paramedic. A paramedic cannot choose the flight response; although I have known it to happen at the scene of a cardiac arrest – needless to say, he joined the dole queue!

A paramedic needs to act fast under any circumstances: Adrenaline can cause you to freeze on the spot, practically glue you to the floor.

A paramedic needs to think on his feet: Oxygen is drawn away from the brain, causing confusion.

A paramedic needs to be able to listen to what is being said: Environmental deafness often occurs.

A paramedic needs to be able to ask questions and give out clear instructions to his crewmate and other emergency services: A dry, pasty mouth can cause a tremor in the voice.

A paramedic needs steady hands to be able to carefully and accurately put a needle into a patient's vein (cannulation), or a tube down their windpipe (intubation): Adrenaline causes the hands to sweat and shake like crazy.

It's bizarre. Here I was, a picture of health – compared to this poor sod anyway, who was absolutely covered in blood – and my body responded as if it was *my* life in danger. Fortunately I understood adrenaline and knew to accept it and control it through diaphragmatic breathing.

Diaphragmatic breathing helps close down the sympathetic nervous system, which is responsible for speeding *things* up in the body. Diaphragmatic breathing shuts off the fear; it switches off the adrenaline release. When you take deep breaths you fool the brain in to thinking that the 'threat' to your life has gone. Obviously there was no threat to me, but like I said, our body perceives even a driving test to be a threat to life. The other very important aspect of understanding adrenaline is learning to hide it; you can't entirely, but it is possible. By doing so, the patient doesn't perceive you to be panicking.

Most people do not understand adrenaline; they view the side effects as fear and then begin to panic. If a patient notices the paramedic panicking then the patient, or the patient's friends or loved ones watching, are likely to begin panicking too, assuming that if the paramedic is panicking, something must be seriously wrong. However, working at speed is not the same as panicking; it is simply recognising that time is of the essence, and understanding that seconds save lives.

Anyway, let's get back to the scene.

When we reached the patient's side, I acknowledged the copper but was immediately drawn to the 'claret' soaking the entire front of the casualty's unzipped bomber jacket and his t-shirt, which was dripping, from his yet to be fully identified wounds, on to the grass. I knelt down next to him, the adrenaline continuing to course through my veins like a steam train; but I'd learnt how to remain calm on the outside, like a duck gliding along the surface of a pond, even though on the inside my heart was going ten to the dozen, like a duck's little webbed feet underwater. I gazed at his face and was astonished by the sheer pallor of his skin; he was grey, sweaty and extremely clammy to the touch. I then looked at his chest, quickly noticing that every time he breathed, his t-shirt concaved inwards while a rapid sucking noise could be heard. So I took a deep breath and, as calmly as possible, began ascertaining some details from him.

'What's y'name, mate?' I asked, trying to hide the little tremor in my voice. His eyes were closed but he opened them when he heard my voice, and muttered what I heard to be Jason, but it sounded incomprehensible. Nevertheless, I was able to assess and confirm his conscious level as 'responds to verbal stimuli'.

In the medical profession, the 'AVPU' scale is used to quickly assess a patient's consciousness level:

'A' is 'Alert'.

'V' is 'responds to Verbal stimuli'.

'P' is 'responds to Painful stimuli'.

'U' is 'Unresponsive to any stimuli'.

Based on his AVPU, I quickly took out a nasopharyngeal airway adjunct (a narrow tube made of soft, malleable plastic) from the paramedic bag, applied KY jelly to it, and inserted it with a twisting motion into his right nostril. This would ensure a patent airway in the event his conscious level reduced further, causing him to be unable to maintain his own airway. The fact that he tolerated a tube inserted into his nose was secondary confirmation that he had a lowered conscious level. I then applied an oxygen mask to his face and administered high flow oxygen to him.

With Adam stood by my side, initially redundant, I took hold of Jason's wrist to feel for a radial pulse, and to check for the rate of his pulse too. The presence of a radial pulse signifies a systolic blood pressure of *at least* eighty millimetres of mercury, or

80mmHg, although textbook figures vary. A normal adult 'textbook' systolic blood pressure would be one hundred and twenty millimetres of mercury, or 120mmHg. A systolic below 90mmHg is considered low blood pressure.

Systolic means the arterial pressure during contraction of the heart. It is measured in 'millimetres of mercury', pertaining to the fact that sphygmomanometers – the equipment used for measuring blood pressure – historically contained mercury, hence the letters 'mmHg' following the preceding figure. The use of mercury sphygmomanometers is no longer common practice amongst health care professionals around the globe, and has generally been replaced with digital instruments, and aneroid types that have a dial. Palpating a radial pulse is merely an approximate measurement prior to actually measuring a patient's blood pressure.

Jason didn't have a palpable radial pulse, so I checked for a central pulse (i.e. the carotid pulse in his neck). He had one. That indicated to me that his systolic blood pressure was at least 60mmHg, but at that level it would be life-threateningly low! Given the absence of a palpable radial pulse, I could only assume – by the state of Jason's car and how he was presenting in my primary 'Airway, Breathing and Circulation' (ABC) survey – that his blood pressure was 'in his boots'. He was in hypovolaemic shock caused by a low volume of blood. His vital organs were not being adequately perfused due to an insufficient amount of oxygenated blood circulating the body. He was shutting down right in front of me and would soon die without invasive action.

I pressed hard on the nail bed of his right hand, which caused Jason to pull away. Then, I rapidly made a mental calculation of his Glasgow Coma Score, or GCS. To keep it really simple, a GCS is a number from three to fifteen based on a patient's consciousness level – which can fluctuate, both up and down, throughout an assessment and treatment. Anything lower than fifteen is classed as a reduced level of consciousness; Jason's GCS was nine. He scored three for responding to my voice, a two for making incomprehensible sounds, and a four for withdrawing from painful stimuli when I pressed hard on the nail bed of his right hand. A GCS of nine was poor to say the least.

Adam was stood beside me, taken aback by Jason's presentation. The copper, still holding Jason's head, looked directly at me,

'What do you want me to do, mate?' he asked, with a look of alarm on his face. Almost simultaneously, Adam gazed at me with a helpless expression and said,

'What do you want mate?' Reality kicked in. I thought where's the paramedic I was used to looking to for support, where is he? He's not here.

My paramedic course flashed before my eyes. I'd practiced critical trauma scenarios countless times just weeks ago; this was now the real thing. I took a couple of deep breaths, right from the bottom of the diaphragm. The trauma knowledge came flooding to the front of my brain, ready to implement. Time was of the essence because Jason had time-critical features, and the outcome would depend on how quick I initiated his assessment and treatment, and got him to a trauma centre.

In a trauma setting there are terms called the Golden Hour and the Platinum Ten. The Golden Hour means that if an unstable patient with time-critical features is being assessed and treated in hospital, preferably a trauma centre, within an hour from the time of the incident, then the prognosis is far better than if they are not in hospital within the hour.

The Platinum Ten is the number of minutes – from arriving at the patient's side to being mobile to hospital – it should preferably take a paramedic to assess and provide initial treatment to a seriously injured trauma patient. It can be done, and was done on numerous occasions during trauma scenarios just several weeks previous, on my paramedic course. However, it's not always that simple in real life as it is in training.

Adam and the copper were awaiting a response.

'Right, you keep holding his head and keep talking to him, that's it!' I said to the copper.

'Adam, you get the scoop stretcher, head-blocks, Velcro straps and a rigid collar. No spider straps! We haven't got time to put the spider straps on. He's time-critical, so we'll have to sacrifice full immobilisation to save his life.' The copper remained where he was, holding Jason's head. Adam ran off towards the ambulance to fetch the equipment I had requested. I pulled out my tuff cut scissors and started cutting Jason's t-shirt off, from the bottom upwards, leaving his unzipped bomber jacket in place. When I reached the top of the t-shirt and opened out the sides and exposed his upper body, there was a huge hole in the right-hand side of his chest, the size of two adult hands. The majority of the right side of his chest and ribcage had been obliterated by a brutal outside force that had barely ripped his t-shirt on impact. I could visibly see his right lung, which had also sustained severe damage.

The sucking noise was caused by a large fold of skin tissue, flapping as environmental air entered and escaped the large space in his chest with each rapid breath. And now the t-shirt was cut open, it became very clear that this young lad was not long for this earth. Adrenaline continued to hurtle through my veins, and the inside of my chest felt like a boxer was using my heart as a speed ball – B'dum-B'dum-B'dum-B'dum-B'dum-B'dum-B'dum-B'dum-B'dum. I'm sure I could hear my own heartbeat over the whistling of the surrounding sparrows. I accepted it was adrenaline and I would not allow it to cause me to panic. It was there to help me get through this ordeal. So, once again I took a couple of deep breaths to fool my brain into believing the threat had gone. I opened up some large ambulance dressings, placing them, unfolded, over the huge, gaping, haemorrhaging chest wound, to keep it as clean as possible.

Again, I asked Jason his name, age and other distracting questions; I hadn't forgotten his name, I was just assessing to see if his AVPU had reduced from a 'V' to a 'P' or a 'U'. I cut the right-hand sleeve of his bomber jacket and applied a tourniquet to his arm, and then began rummaging through the paramedic bag for a cannula; a needle that you insert into a vein, leaving a clear plastic tube in place to administer drugs or fluids, or sometimes both. I chose the largest diameter cannula that paramedics carry; it is a wide needle, primarily used for life-threatening trauma injuries, and it was safe to say that it was a good time to use one. Jason was so shut down that even the tourniquet was not engorging any veins in his arm.

With my heart still going like the clappers, I took several deep breaths to try and control the adrenaline from causing my hands to shake. I patted his arm where a vein should physiologically be and pierced the skin with the needle, practically cannulating blindfold. Jason tried to pull his arm away when the needle pierced his skin, but I was restraining his arm for that very reason. I was praying for blood to appear in the flashback chamber, which usually confirms successful intravenous access. The flashback appeared, so I advanced the needle further and awaited a secondary flashback to appear along the length of the clear plastic tube. The secondary flashback appeared.

'Nice one, I'm in,' I said to the copper, followed by a deep sigh of relief.

With an evident flashback, I unclipped the tourniquet, applied digital (thumb) pressure to the vein, withdrew the needle and discarded the needle into the sharps container, leaving the clear plastic tube inside his vein. I screwed the Luer-Lock to the end and quickly secured it in place with an adhesive dressing, before flushing it with a pre-filled, ten-millilitre syringe of sodium chloride to confirm patent 'IV access' – he was going to need it!

With 'IV access' secured, I turned to the copper,

'What 'appened 'ere anyway?' I asked with my mind racing, waiting for Adam to return. 'And why is he so far away from the car?'

'The bloke over there witnessed it. He said he lost control on the bend, crashed through the fence, and then crashed into that tree. So he ran over and pulled him out of the car and laid him here. A piece of timber smashed through the windscreen and staked his chest,' the copper explained.

'Bloody 'ell,' I said, shaking my head with disbelief that he was still alive.

Adam returned with the equipment. He positioned the scoop on to the ground, separated it and placed one half either side of Jason. That's the beauty of the scoop, it separates in two, and then each part can be slid underneath the patient and clipped back together, forming a stretcher. With the copper still immobilising Jason's head, I placed the collar around his neck, then with Adam used a synchronised rolling method and positioned each half of the scoop underneath Jason, before clipping the two ends together. I then put a head-block on each side of his head and secured them in place with Velcro straps. As we were doing that, much to my relief, Danny, an experienced paramedic in an RRV (Rapid Response Vehicle) rolled up on blue lights. I wasn't looking to him for advice – I was coping well – so before he even had chance to place one foot on the grass, I turned and stared at him with what must have looked like madman eyes, and shouted,

'Danny, get me a litre of fluid set up, now!'

He immediately, without hesitation, leapt on to our ambulance and began to set up the bag of fluid I had less than politely requested. The fluid I was going to use – sodium chloride – doesn't have oxygen carrying capabilities like blood has, it merely increases the volume of fluid in the body's circulatory system. Nonetheless, it can improve the prognosis in a hypovolaemic patient.

As we had now placed Jason onto the scoop stretcher, we then, between me, Adam and the copper, lifted him across the twenty-five yards of the field to the ambulance and placed the scoop onto the ambulance stretcher. I quickly attached the fluid administration equipment that Danny had prepared, known as a 'fluid giving set', to the cannula in Jason's arm and opened up the clamp so fluid would run rapidly through his veins. This was intended to increase his blood pressure to the point he had a palpable radial pulse, thus confirming a systolic blood pressure of at least 80mmHg. However, as the body has a natural defence mechanism to clot haemorrhaging, administering fluid can encourage clots to dilute and break down, therefore causing haemorrhaging to recommence – if haemorrhaging has ceased – or it can reduce the body's own natural clotting factors from functioning. That was a consideration I had to take into account when I opened up the clamp and infused fluid into Jason. I didn't have a lot of choice though. His blood pressure was so low that he would die without, what we call in the medical profession, a 'fluid challenge'.

'Right, Adam, get on to ambulance control and tell 'em to alert A 'n' E. I want a full trauma team including anaesthetist. Tell 'em RTC versus fence and tree, in that order. Driver nineteen years old, GCS nine, open sucking chest wound. Tell 'em to request 'O' negative blood t'be on standby. Do it now!' I said, with clear instruction in my voice.

'OK mate,' Adam replied.

I felt for a palpable radial pulse again; he still didn't have one. I wasn't expecting one yet, I was just being impatient, so I allowed the fluid to keep draining from the hanging drip into his veins. I shone my pen torch into each of his pupils to assess that they were both equal in size and reactive to light. That does not necessarily rule out a head injury, but is a positive sign if the pupils are equal and reactive to light. Fortunately, Jason's pupils were normal, but based on the state of his car crunched against the tree, a head injury could not be ruled out, yet.

While periodically feeling for a radial pulse in his wrist, I continued to cut off the rest of his clothes, from his socks and trainers upwards, in order to completely expose his body, with the exception of his underwear for dignity purposes. When I started cutting the body of the bomber jacket off, it became apparent that it was filled with feathers, and because of the breeze flowing through the open rear doors of the ambulance, the feathers went everywhere; floating around the saloon, landing in his open wounds, landing in the blood on his body and into the blood that had dripped on to the floor from his open chest wound and other less serious haemorrhaging injuries. I needed the jacket off though, to expose the whole of his upper body so the doctors could undertake a rapid secondary survey; that is look, listen and feel for other injuries on the body in addition to the obvious injuries he had. Then I covered him with several blankets to keep him warm, as he was by now practically as naked as the day he was born.

Adam had conveyed a pre-alert message to the ambulance dispatcher, who would pass on the information to the receiving hospital's A&E department. He then closed the rear and side doors, adopted his position in the driver's seat and began mobilising on blue lights to hospital, which was only a few miles away. I took hold of Jason's wrist and felt for a palpable radial pulse. He still didn't have one.

'Bloody 'ell, he's lost a bucket full,' I thought. I gazed at his chest as the wound continued to make a sucking sound every time he breathed in and out. Then, all of a sudden, Jason spoke,

'Am I gonna die?' He paused momentarily. 'Am I gonna die? I've gotta girlfriend,' he mumbled, at the same time opened his eyes.

'You just keep talkin' to me Jason, you're gonna be fine,' I said, attempting to reassure him. 'Your name is Jason, isn't it?'

'Uh... think,' he confusedly muttered. I didn't know what else to say. I couldn't exactly reply with yes, probably mate, you've got bloody awful injuries so there's very little chance you're going to survive... could I! However, because he had asked me a question with his eyes open, without any verbal or painful stimuli from me, meant that his GCS had increased from nine to twelve; probably due to the IV fluid and oxygen I'd administered having a positive effect on his circulation, thus causing more oxygenated blood to travel to his brain. By now, 800 millilitres of fluid had infused through the cannula in his arm. So I felt for a radial pulse again, and there was one; excellent I thought. It was weak but nonetheless palpable. The fluid had worked. It had increased his blood pressure to a level adequate enough to buy him time for the real lifesavers to go to work on him. I adjusted the clamp so the fluid infusion reduced to a very steady drip, because I didn't want to increase his blood pressure too much.

Throughout the journey to hospital, all I did was periodically monitor the amount of fluid draining from the hanging drip, and hold his wrist to make sure he maintained a radial pulse and to give him some assurance that someone was there with him. I didn't measure his oxygen saturations, better known as *sats* or *SP02*, which is a measurement of how well oxygenated the blood is in the body. I didn't undertake a single measurement of his blood pressure, blood glucose or even analyse an ECG to see what his exact heart rate and rhythm was. It didn't matter. This guy needed doctors; an A&E consultant, an anaesthetist and a surgeon to be precise, not a paramedic playing around on scene, ticking all the boxes to meet the criteria for pre-hospital trauma found in a textbook. The basic paramedic skill of high flow oxygen administration, a cannula and a fluid challenge was keeping him alive.

As we approached the hospital, I reassured Jason that we were nearly there; by 'there' I meant the place he needed to be if he stood any chance of survival, although I obviously didn't say that to him. When we eventually arrived at A&E – it felt like a lifetime even though it had only been several minutes – Adam parked up in the ambulance bay, vacated his seat, and quickly opened the rear doors and lowered the ramp. A trauma team had gathered in the entrance doorway, awaiting the patient they had been put on alert for; they were all gloved and gowned ready to pounce on the poor sod. We wheeled the stretcher inside and quickly lifted the scoop onto the resuscitation bed.

The room was by now swarming with medical staff, and an appointed lead doctor was awaiting my handover. As paramedics are usually the first health care professionals on scene and hold vital information about an incident, a doctor usually listens to a handover from the paramedic while other doctors commence the assessment and treatment of the sick or injured patient. In this case, for instance, information on the extent of the damage to the vehicle, what the approximate speed of impact was, and what injuries have been sustained, to name but a few. A handover is intended to summarise the history of events and observations undertaken by the paramedic, and the treatment provided. A handover is not usually conveyed grammatically or in full sentences, because doing so prolongs the process; if you have requested the resuscitation room, then the doctor needs information fast! Therefore, a handover is usually passed without interruption from anyone else in the resuscitation room.

I must emphasise that handovers do not always flow in as structured a way as you would like them to. Sometimes you forget some of the information that would be beneficial to the A&E consultant, due to the extent of the observations ascertained and the treatment you have provided. It is an acquired skill, and I'm not afraid to admit that I'm still trying to improve my handover technique to the present day.

For the benefit of the layperson, I have simplified handovers throughout this book. Therefore my handover went something like this:

'Right, this is Jason. Approximately nineteen years old. Jason was a single occupant of a Subaru driving approximately sixty mile per hour. Jason crashed through a fence; sudden halt on impact with a large tree trunk at 0650 hours. Seatbelt worn.

'Jason was pulled from the car by a bystander. On arrival he was lay flat on his back and a police officer was immobilising c-spine. Airway patent but nasal airway inserted and tolerated. AVPU initially V. GCS initially nine, but increased to twelve on route. Rapid shallow respiratory rate, O2 administered. No initial palpable radial pulse. He was grey, sweaty and clammy.

'On examination, huge open, sucking chest wound caused by a wooden stake through the windscreen; which I've covered as best as I could. Mechanism of injury cannot rule out spinal, pelvic or head injury. Pupils equal and reactive to light.

'No sats. No blood pressure. No blood glucose. No ECG monitored, and only partial immobilisation applied due to him presenting with life-threatening, time-critical features. Patient's clothes cut off but no opportunity to do secondary survey.

'Large bore IV cannula inserted into the right arm, and just over eight hundred millilitres of fluid administered to restore a palpable radial pulse, which I have confirmed as present on route and on arrival here at A&E.

'Are there any questions?'

'No, thank you... well done,' the doctor replied, looking alternately between me and Jason.

Within a few minutes of arriving at A&E, Jason had been anaesthetised, intubated and manually ventilated by the anaesthetist. He was also catheterised, had another large bore cannula inserted into his left arm, his blood pressure and blood glucose measured, and had also been attached to an ECG monitor. He was in good hands and plenty of them.

It's amazing what can be done when there are more than two medical professionals available to attempt to stabilise a dying patient. All I had done was keep his blood pressure up with IV fluid, which bought him valuable time, and then scoop and run to the nearest hospital. The incident had gone smooth, and we had achieved the Golden Hour and the Platinum Ten too.

Adam and I then went outside to deeply inhale some much needed air, leaving the doctors to work on trying to stabilise Jason. We both gazed into the back of the ambulance through the open rear doors; it was an absolute mess, with feathers, equipment, packaging and blood everywhere, on the floor, up the walls, on the cupboard doors. It looked like ten chickens had been slaughtered. I looked down at my uniform to find more blood on me than an abattoir's floor; I'd paid no attention to how blood-soiled I'd become while treating Jason.

I started the paperwork while Adam had an attempt at cleaning up the mess in the ambulance to restore it to an acceptable standard, prior to its inevitable deep clean by a private, infection control valeting company. There was no doubt that it was coming off the road and out of service for the rest of the day.

We should have finished our shift at 7 a.m. but we only cleared from hospital at 9 a.m. Once my paperwork was complete, the ambulance clean (cleanish anyway), and our job done, we headed on back to the station. Throughout the twenty minute journey, we barely said a word to each other, probably due to tiredness of what was now becoming nearly a fifteen hour non-stop shift; and also because we were both still a little stunned from what we had just experienced.

When we arrived back at the station there was nobody about. We had taken so long at hospital, completing paperwork and cleaning the ambulance, that our relief crew had taken a spare ambulance and gone out on stand-by, or to a treble-nine or urgent call. Adam and I went into the changing room and carefully removed our blood-stained uniforms, being careful not to touch the claret-soaked areas, and then placed the lot into a clinical waste bag, ready for the furnace. There was no point in trying to salvage uniform; we had plenty of it for incidents that involved getting covered in excessive bodily fluids. We scrubbed up, put our 'civvies' on, had a quick chat and then went our separate ways to our awaiting beds.

By the time I arrived home, I had been awake for so long that I'd started getting a second stamina and didn't want to go to bed. So I sat on the couch with a cup of tea, reminiscing over the job. It suddenly dawned on me why Mr X – my paramedic instructor – had been so relentless; it was necessary in order to cope with incidents like the one Adam and I had just dealt with. And without all that intense training, study and all those character testing fictitious scenarios, I honestly don't think I'd have been able to handle it, let alone take charge.

Later that night, back on night shift duty, after I'd handed over a patient to the nurse in A&E, I asked the A&E consultant who had cared for Jason what had happened to him. He informed me that he remained in a critical condition and had been transferred to the Cardiothoracic Centre later that day, where both in and out-patients go for heart (cardio) and chest (thoracic) related diagnosis, treatment or surgery.

I very rarely went to the Cardiothoracic Centre, so was unable to find out what happened to Jason. It is often very difficult for paramedics to follow-up their patients' diagnosis, continuing treatment or outcome once they have been handed over to A&E. Patients are either admitted to a ward, discharged or, like Jason, transferred to another hospital, and you cannot just ring up the hospital and ask how a patient is doing, because you could be anyone. They won't just take your word for it that you're the paramedic who dealt with a particular patient you're enquiring about.

However, six months later I conveyed an elderly patient to the Cardiothoracic Centre for a routine out-patient appointment. So, while I was there, I couldn't resist the temptation to ask the receptionist if she could check on the patient data system for information if I gave her Jason's full name, which I had remembered with ease, and although not strictly permissible, she obliged. I also gave her some background information as to what had happened and what injuries Jason had sustained on that adrenal-fuelled morning. The receptionist, shocked and intrigued at the story, browsed the system for his details. I waited in anticipation, and after a bit of swift keyboard tapping, she found his records.

'Did he make it? Did he survive?' I asked impatiently, leaning over the reception desk. She looked up at me and smiled,

'Yeah, he's been discharged and has a routine follow-up appointment in six months.'

'No way! That's excellent, nice one!' I replied, with a beaming grin on my face.

I couldn't believe it. With the injuries he had sustained, nobody would have believed he could have possibly survived long enough for surgeons to go to work on him, but by some miracle he had. Although he would have to live with *huge* physical scars – and no doubt mental scars too – that would remind him of that very day and those horrendous injuries that he sustained, for the rest of his life.

Chapter 2
A Thousand Mile Journey

Since experiencing my *Baptism of Fire*, I have attended to hundreds upon hundreds of traumatic incidents as the lead clinician – the paramedic. Those incidents include further road traffic collisions, railway incidents, light aircraft crashes, falls from a significant height, stabbings, shootings, severe burns and many more, some of which inevitably involved fatalities. But how did I come to arrive at the unpredictable door of The Dark Side, where not only is every shift different, but also where all of the incidents I have written about in this book would become experiences I will never forget for the rest of my life?

I guess it all started when I left secondary school in 1992 and began working. Having a keen interest in physical fitness training, fighting arts and self-defence from the start of secondary school to the present day, I chose to spend the majority of my early working life in the leisure and fitness industry, as a qualified pool lifeguard, fitness instructor and self-employed personal fitness trainer. With the exception of a few other jobs, that occupied me up until June 2002, when I commenced employment with the NHS Ambulance Service.

During my career as a fitness trainer, both employed and self-employed, I regularly undertook consultations on clients who had paid their hard-earned cash to lose fat and get fit, amongst other reasons of course. During consultations, clients would confide in me about their medical ailments, illnesses, medications and occasionally their personal problems too (I won't go in to them stories!). I would frequently hear medical terms no layperson would believe existed, so would therefore have to regularly research and educate myself about numerous medical conditions in order to prescribe an appropriate, effective and safe exercise programme for the client; not only so they would achieve their

23

aims, but also so I didn't contribute towards their death! It may be funny on *You've Been Framed* watching some poor sod fall flat on his face on a treadmill, and then involuntarily fly backwards with a towel around his shoulders, as if rewinding a *Superman* DVD, but in real life it's not a pleasant sight at all, I can assure you; especially when they fall off the treadmill due to suffering a heart attack!

Over a period of time I became progressively more interested in anatomy and physiology, medical conditions and the medical profession in general. I'd often thought to myself I'd love to be a paramedic, dealing with car crashes, heart attacks, making a difference to people when they're sick, injured or in pain, or maybe even save someone's life. Unfortunately though, I'd only left school with a handful of GCSEs; with poor grades, I reluctantly add. I therefore lacked the qualifications and grades that I needed to achieve a paramedical career.

Nevertheless, and regardless of the fact that I hadn't pursued a medical career, I did eventually make the decision that a long-term career as a fitness instructor was not for me. So, in the summer of 1998, I left employment in the gym facility I was working at but continued to work as a self-employed personal fitness trainer, and also secured employment with Royal Mail as a postman. Becoming a postman was an unusual career deviation I know, but I wanted more time to physically train myself. Being a postman gave me ample opportunity to do just that.

Fast forward almost two years, and I had still made no progression towards a medical career whatsoever. However, while I was strolling along delivering mail one spring morning in the year of 2000, I once again began pondering over my long-term future. It occurred to me that there was such an establishment called college, a place where second chances are an option for under-achievers like me. I thought hard about my interest in anatomy and physiology and the medical profession, particularly the paramedical profession, and thought maybe I *could* become a paramedic. I may not be the most studious of people but I was quite knowledgeable when it came to the human body and medical conditions, although it didn't take me long before I began feeling negative about my overambitious thoughts.

'What chance have I got of becoming a paramedic?' I asked myself repeatedly. 'I'm just a postman. Postmen don't become paramedics. Paramedics save lives; that can't be easy,' I thought, with the self-doubt that I, uneducated me, could achieve such a feat. I continued along, delivering letters and parcels, and a few streets later and a much lighter sack of mail over my shoulder, I had slowly but surely begun convincing myself that I could do it, it was within my league of possible achievements.

So I started thinking hard about what I would have to do to even apply for the Ambulance Service, let alone get accepted. I would have to go back to college to prove on paper that I was capable of *Reading, Riting and Rithmetic* (I've never understood that term!). I would also have to save a lot of money to fund the driver training needed to obtain categories C1 and D1 on my driving licence; due to changes in law, I didn't automatically gain categories C1 and D1 when I passed my driving test. Those categories were a prerequisite to even apply for the Ambulance Service back then, and still are today, I think. I know category C1 is definitely a requirement, as most UK ambulances have a gross weight over seven and a half ton.

With all that in mind I thought right, that's it, I'm going to begin putting my plans into action; I was capable of a lot more than simply posting mail for the rest of my working life. My mind was inquisitive; it needed challenging, stimulating... regularly! Being a postman seldom did that, if ever. I was also getting bored of listening to the same old,

'If it's a bill, mate, you can keep it,' and 'It's a good job, postman, isn't it? Better than walking the streets, hey!' It's funny at first but it wears a little thin hearing it umpteen times a day, six days a week, week in week out. I was also becoming intolerant of being stopped by youngsters a mile away from their postal address and asking me for their giro, and when I'd refuse to give it to them (by law), they'd blatantly inform me that they wanted it there and then so they could cash it on their way home from work; the bloody nerve of the cheeky little scrotes! I can't even call them work-shy cheeky little scrotes.

I began making enquiries by doing some extensive research. I contacted the local College of Further Education with reference to adult access courses, and also requested an information pack from the Ambulance Service Human Resources department, which arrived within a few days of my request. I perused the literature with mixed emotions: confusion, excitement and apprehension. Nevertheless, I wasn't deterred; in fact I was even more determined than ever. I'd digested the information and was ready and willing to begin the journey from Postman to Paramedic.

'A thousand mile journey begins with the first step,' I thought. At that point I reckon I had about 999 miles left to endure, which was apt.

So I ceased self-employment and enrolled on a college course for mature students, and started in September 2000. The course enabled me to prove on paper that I could read, write and apply basic arithmetic. The timetable gave me the opportunity to blitz my *walk* (delivery route), get home, get showered, have a bite to eat and get to college on time for class. The downside to the timetable was that there were morning classes, sometimes nothing in the afternoons, and then evening lessons, which prolonged the day and proved to be very tiring.

During the early stages of the course, I went that extra mile and joined the Institute of Advanced Motorists (IAM) and, after ten or so ninety-minute sessions with an IAM observer, and a two hour driving test examined by a class one traffic cop, I was awarded my advanced driving certificate. The advanced driving qualification was intended to be an added bonus to my application form, to earn some 'Brownie points' with the short-listing panel. I also hoped it would improve my chances of passing the strict driving test element of the selection process too.

I persevered with the college course and the mundane routine day in, day out. I'd get up at 4 a.m., eat, go to the sorting office, sort my mail, walk around delivering mail for several hours, get home, get showered, eat, drive to college, sit through a mathematics class, drive home, eat, go back to college for an English class, drive home again and, well… have something to eat, of course; well an empty bin-bag won't stand up, will it! Once I was fed and watered, I'd go to bed about 11 p.m. and cop myself some Z's until 4 a.m., when I would do it all over again. It was tough going but I was hell bent on success.

In June 2001, having finished the course and attained significantly improved GCSE grades, I continued striving to achieve my career ambition by working myself into the ground to fund the extortionate fees to obtain categories C1 and D1 on my driving licence. While still working as a postman, I signed up to temping agencies and accepted two-ten shifts in factories, packing boxes, picking orders, and believe it or not, removing unusable peanuts from a moving carousel, and other mind-numbingly boring jobs. Those types of jobs are not good for the mind; brain cells die doing monotonous jobs like that, I'm certain.

I remember a colleague of mine at the sorting office telling me that, before he joined Royal Mail, he had worked in a plastics factory that manufactured and distributed buckets. He explained to me what the manager, who had provided the 'training', had said to him on his first day. He said,

'You take hold of a bucket… then take hold of a handle… and then you put the handle on the bucket.' Well I nearly pissed myself laughing, not because of the job itself, but because the job was deemed to need 'training'. I'm sure the manager could have got away with saying, 'Put a handle on each bucket, simple!' I remember saying to my colleague, after I'd emptied my bladder of course, having nearly pissed my pants,

'You should have frowned and replied I don't understand chief, can you run that by me again?'

I'm not making fun; I actually have a lot of respect and admiration for those that stick it in dead-end jobs like that their whole lives, because I simply couldn't do it. Although I did last longer than my colleague; he only lasted fifty-two minutes in that factory putting buckets on handles – I mean handles on buckets. Oh, whatever!

I could have taken up personal training again, but to be honest I'd lost the passion that was expected of me from the clients who would be paying good money for me to help them achieve their personal goals. My energy and passion was entirely focused on a career in the Ambulance Service, and I was determined to achieve a vocation where I would have to use my brain and be paid from the neck up, and not from the neck down.

I slogged away doing an abundance of brain-cell-destroying temping jobs, and before I knew it I had enough money to pay for the pre-requisite intensive driving courses. I passed my Class 2 HGV driving test in the October of 2001, which meant I automatically obtained category C1. And in February 2002 I obtained my category D1 licence. With both pre-requisite driving categories under my belt, and my improved GCSE grades, I'd finally met the minimum criteria to apply for the Patient Transport Service (PTS), and it just so happened that Mersey Regional Ambulance Service were recruiting. Perfect timing or what! I was still nowhere near becoming a paramedic, but if I could just get into the PTS, I would be going in the right direction and well on my way to achieving my goal.

For those that don't know what the PTS is, it is the non-emergency aspect of the NHS Ambulance Service. The main purpose of the role is to pick up the old dears from their homes and convey them to their out-patient appointments, wait for them, and then take them home again. Basic and boring it may sound, but the experience one gains from working in the PTS sets the foundations and fundamental skills required to progress further up the ladder in the ambulance service. For example, patient care, communication, dealing with the public, 'bedside' manner, geographical knowledge, and various conveyance routes to a number of regional hospitals, to name but a few.

It was common amongst ambulance staff to discuss the benefits of several months on PTS before becoming an ambulance technician; and with the exception of a handful of staff, it was very easy to single out those who joined the service direct as ambulance technicians, having never experienced the benefits of the PTS role. Even to this day, I still benefit from the experience I gained starting out my career on the PTS. I kid you not, it was invaluable. In fact, I think it should be compulsory for anyone wanting to be a paramedic. I know from past conversations that others share the same opinion too.

In June 2002, after spending several months periodically and successfully completing various selection tests for the PTS – application form, theory, driving, fitness and medical tests, interview, criminal records bureau and references – I was accepted into the PTS and subsequently resigned from Royal Mail, admittedly with a little apprehension. I was apprehensive because at the time, working for Royal Mail was considered a redundant-proof job; it kept you fit, the camaraderie was fantastic, and your customers appreciated you – most of them, anyway. And there was very little danger involved when compared to the potential dangers faced by ambulance personnel. The only real dangers of being a postman were dogs, particularly the ankle biting type – I hate ankle biters, give me a Rottweiler over a Jack Russell any day.

There was also the occasional malicious drug addict (potentially HIV positive) who would Blu-Tack a used needle inside the letterbox, so the postman's hand got needle-sticked when they pushed the mail through. That nasty act genuinely occurred on some estates, particularly those estates that made Beirut look like Dubai – the estates I delivered to. Fortunately though, it never happened to me, *but* had it I'd have been fine, as I always took precaution before posting mail through a druggie's door... I always put a condom on!

So I left Royal Mail and began my ambulance service career, which started with one week's classroom tuition, learning how to correctly lift patients down a flight of stairs using the carry chair; basic first-aid including oxygen administration; map reading; and how to fold blankets and correctly wrap a blanket around a patient in such a way that Florence Nightingale would have been impressed (not). Then one week's driver training, followed by ten months' experience gaining the fundamental, yet vital skills I would need to progress further on my mission to become a professional paramedic.

Around March 2003, the opportunity to apply for Ambulance Technician training came along. As previously mentioned, an Ambulance Technician is a paramedic's assistant, a lesser skilled and qualified member of ambulance personnel. However, it was common for two technicians to work together; not ideal, but several years ago there was a shortage of qualified paramedics, and there still is today, I am led to believe. Back then, technician training and at least twelve months' experience was compulsory if you endeavoured to apply for paramedic training.

For a further several months I had to endure additional theory, practical, fitness and medical tests, and also a further interview in front of a panel of managers. A short time after I had completed the various stages of selection, the news I'd anxiously been waiting for finally came via a telephone call from my PTS manager. She informed me that I had been selected from two thousand applicants for just ten Ambulance Technician vacancies. I was finally transferring to The Dark Side. Years of hard work, sleep deprivation and several additional mundane jobs had finally begun paying off; and as you can imagine, I was absolutely ecstatic.

I began the ten week intensive Ambulance Technician course with nine others, several of them my peers from the PTS; the others were direct entrants from the street. The course consisted of two weeks' emergency driver training – or three weeks for the direct entrants – and eight weeks' intense theoretical, practical and scenario-based training, with frequent pass or fail examinations. Candidates were taught anatomy and physiology; how to manage respiratory, cardiac, diabetic, epileptic and trauma patients; how to interpret basic ECG heart rhythms; Basic Life Support (CPR); how and when to administer specific 'technician' drugs; the preparation of 'drips' and intravenous drugs for paramedics to administer, and much more.

Upon me successfully completing the course, then followed twelve months' experience under the supervision of a paramedic, or sometimes a more experienced technician. In order to fully qualify as an Institute of Health Care and Development (IHCD) Ambulance Technician, a specific portfolio had to be completed and signed off by an appropriately trained mentor, and then verified by the IHCD. Although tough going, my twelve month probationary technician period was absolutely fantastic. The station life, the camaraderie, the learning that took place, the scenes, the humour and the experiences were all amazing – not all pleasant, granted, but nevertheless amazing – and would prove not only to be essential to my development as a technician but also to me becoming a professional paramedic.

After approximately fourteen months as an Ambulance Technician, and having gained a great deal of knowledge and experience, I was asked by the Station Manager if I would like to attempt paramedic selection. I remember a comment from a colleague of mine, an exceptional paramedic, one I aspired to be like one day. He said,

'Andy, you're ready for your paras, mate. You know when you're ready for your paras when you think exactly what the paramedic you're working with is thinking. You do what he is going to tell you to do, before he even tells you to do it; and you start preparing the drug you know he is going to ask you for, and the exact dosage appropriate for the patient. You're ready mate.' With that comment in mind, I told the Station Manager that I'd be delighted to attempt paramedic selection; as if I was going to say no!

Again I had to undergo more theory and practical examinations, and another interview, with just one manager this time, not a panel. And to my relief, I was quickly informed that I had been selected for the next course. I was delighted. I was actually getting closer and closer to achieving the ambition I had been pursuing since contemplating my future as a postman several years previous. The same ambition I told myself that *I*, uneducated me, could not achieve.

The paramedic course consisted of eight weeks' intense theoretical, practical and scenario-based training, again with frequent pass or fail examinations. The course covered subjects such as more in-depth anatomy and physiology, and advanced cardiac life support (advanced CPR) for adults, paediatrics and neonates; also maternity, cardiac, respiratory, diabetic, epileptic and trauma emergencies. And if that wasn't enough, we were also taught airway management, intravenous access and drug administration, including the pharmacodynamics and pharmacokinetics of a wide variety of drugs, which means what drugs do to the body, and what the body does to drugs. And much, much more.

Then followed one week's placement in the Accident and Emergency (A&E) department of a regional hospital, in order to perform as many intravenous cannulations as possible; one week in the Cardiac Care Unit (CCU), to gain further knowledge of a wide variety of ECG heart rhythms and how to interpret them; and also two weeks in the operating theatres, where we had to successfully put a tube down the airway of twenty-five patients who were 'going under', in order to ventilate them. The four weeks' in-hospital placements were a lot more relaxed, as there wasn't really any theoretical learning involved, only practical learning.

The typical dropout rate during a Mersey Regional Ambulance Service Paramedic Course was between thirty and fifty percent, especially when the instructor, who I shall name Mr X, was an instructor on the course; and it just so happened that Mr X was one of several instructors on my course. I specifically remember the first day of training, and Mr X gave the class a welcome speech which started with,

'Do you all realise what you've let yourselves in for? The next eight weeks are going to be hell.' Excellent, bring it on, I thought. Well there's no growth in comfort, is there!

Although I was very keen, the course proved to be extremely mentally and physically demanding, even more so as I chose to commute on a daily basis to and from the course venue, which was twenty miles from my home. All of the other candidates opted for hotel accommodation from Monday to Friday, for eight weeks, paid for by the NHS Trust. They would go home for the weekend and check-in at the hotel again on the Monday, only to find themselves in a different room, on a different floor. *Forget that!* I thought; I'd rather drive twenty miles twice a day, all week, than choose to mess about like that.

The only downside to commuting was that while them lot were giving it the Z's, my clock would be rudely awakening me at 5 a.m. in order to do a three mile run. Running strengthened my mind and body, ready for another day of learning. I'd leave the house about 7 a.m. in order to miss the rush-hour traffic, and arrive at the venue for around 7:45 a.m. And because I arrived so early, I would be charged with checking that all of the paramedic equipment was in good order, ready for scenario training. Once the checks were complete, I would then indulge in a little airway management practice on the mannequin while waiting for the other candidates to arrive.

Each day the training would commence around 8:45 a.m. In the morning we would sit through lectures. Some of us would endure advanced cardiac life support practical scenarios, have a group debrief, then a tea break, partake in some self-study, and then stop for lunch, which was usually a buffet laid on by the Trust caterers. In the afternoon, with our minds now becoming fatigued by information overload, candidates would endure further lectures, more practical scenarios, and an occasional tea break before the day's training came to a halt at about 5 p.m.; although, on most weekdays throughout the eight weeks of in-house training, several of us would stay behind and put each other through more clinical scenarios, for added practice and confidence building. About 6 p.m., I would drive the twenty miles home and walk through the front door about 6:45 p.m. I'd have my tea, spend a little time with my family, relax a little – very little – before putting my head back in the books until 11 p.m.

That was the Monday to Friday routine. At weekends I'd have a modest lie in, and have two days off from running, and then study practically non-stop from 10 a.m. 'til 5 p.m. That repetitive routine lasted for the full eight weeks, with a risk of exam failure possible at any stage. Throughout the course I barely saw my family, as I was so busy studying that my mind would not allow me to think about hardly anything but clinical practice, including upcoming examinations that I had to pass in order to achieve my ambition. The pressure was constant, but would ultimately pay dividends.

My wife and I still very occasionally reminisce and laugh about the particularly unusual behaviour I revealed during the course, due to me eating, sleeping and… well, you know the saying, paramedical theory and practice. For instance, we both lay in bed one night and, while I was asleep, I subconsciously took hold of her arm, which woke her up. I then straightened her arm out and began tapping on the veins of her arm, and started uttering, as if attending to a time-critical patient,

'That's a good vein. I'll go for that one. Pass me a cannula, quick!'

On another occasion, also while I was asleep, my wife heard me explaining the cardiovascular system in meticulous detail, as if writing an examination essay. Oh my mind was troubled, but it was funny.

Course failure was generally caused by sub-standard knowledge and skill, leading to inadequate exam results, both theoretical and practical. The pass mark for theoretical examinations was eighty-five percent. The practical examinations, which were examined by an external assessor, usually a Resuscitation Officer or a Consultant Anaesthetist, had to be almost faultless. Not easy when you're only human.

I passed all examinations with flying-colours throughout the entire course, with the exception of one. I got eighty-four percent on a trauma paper, and I still remember one of the frustratingly ambiguous questions that I got wrong, that made the difference between getting eighty-four percent and eighty-five percent. I'll tell you what the question was, but if you're a layperson reading this, you may not understand it. Here goes.

Question: Chest trauma will impair internal respiration – true or false?

I chose true. Of course chest trauma will impair internal respiration I thought, during the one-hundred question examination paper. The reason I have never forgotten that question is because it potentially came between me achieving and not achieving my long-term goal; a goal I had spent the last several years chasing with all my passion… and enough blood, sweat and tears spilled to fill an oil-drum. I had just one more chance at a different 'trauma' examination paper, the following day. If I didn't achieve at least eighty-five percent, I would be out, off the course, and would return to technician duties for the foreseeable future.

I went home that night absolutely devastated that I'd come so far and, for the sake of one stupid, ambiguous question, it could all be over. I revised pre-hospital trauma literature practically non-stop until the early hours of the morning, and allowed myself just a couple of hours sleep. Counter-productive, you could say, if I was going to be too tired to concentrate during the upcoming re-sit I would take later that day.

That afternoon, myself and three other candidates who had failed the same paper as me, took our seats in the classroom. Our place on the remainder of the course was down to the next sixty minutes.

'You may begin,' Mr X said. I plugged away for the next hour, reading each question carefully, occasionally becoming frustrated because of the ambiguity. I wanted to shout out *what the feck is that supposed to mean, it could be any one of the four answers?!* But I refrained. For the whole hour the room was incredibly quiet because of the sheer concentration of the candidates; so quiet that you could have heard a pin drop. I could hear the clock ticking away, tick-tock, tick-tock, tick-tock, and before I knew it, Mr X said,

'Stop now, please.' It was an hour that felt like fifteen minutes. Now all I had to do was wait for Mr X to mark it. My future was hanging in the balance. If I didn't pass, I wouldn't even see the day's training out. I'd be driving home immediately, leaving behind the remaining candidates, and be remembered as the fourth, fifth, sixth or seventh candidate to leave the course since it had begun seven weeks previous, depending on how the other three had got on with the exam, that is. Fortunately, we all passed with over eighty-five percent and so remained on the course. Phew!

Now that the four of us had re-sat the examination and had passed, we were able to discuss some of the questions with Mr X. We couldn't discuss any of them immediately after we had failed because some of the same questions from the previous exam would, without a doubt, be in the re-sit exam. So during discussions, the question about chest trauma impairing internal respiration was raised. Mr X informed us that the answer was in fact 'false'; apparently, chest trauma will not impair internal respiration. But – and this is what really annoyed me, because it cost me a clean sweep of exam passes – the full answer was 'False. Chest trauma will not impair internal respiration, but it will eventually'.

'So, the answer to the question is 'true' then?' I said to Mr X.

'No,' he replied.

'But you've just said it will eventually,' I reminded him.

'It will,' he declared, with an expression on his face that said he has a point; it is a silly, ambiguous question. 'But I had to mark you down,' he said.

'That's pathetic! Who writes these exam papers? They need hanging!' I abruptly told Mr X.

There were other reasons, in addition to examination failure, why people left the programme. In some instances, candidates were simply unable to cope with the intense pressure a Mersey Regional Ambulance Service Paramedic Course was notorious for, and would voluntarily leave and return to technician duties for good, with no intention of progressing to paramedic status, ever. An alternative option for referred candidates would be to wait until the opportunity to try the course again was offered to them by management; although that was usually some considerable time later, and not something Mr X was keen to allow without serious consideration. He was passionate about the paramedical profession and didn't want candidates with poor clinical knowledge and practice getting through the course by fluke. He would rather they remained as technicians forever, or until they could prove that they were absolutely capable and ready to be a paramedic, and one with personal high standards of clinical practice too.

He and I didn't always see eye to eye though. I was stubborn when it came to justifying my clinical actions during a medical or trauma scenario. Scenarios were quite realistic, but they were not based on the bread and butter type incidents a paramedic would find themselves attending to on a day-to-day basis, and rightly so! They were designed not only to test your clinical knowledge and skills, but also to test your character under the intense pressure a career as a paramedic often brings.

Scenarios would start with a fictitious patient, with varied or specific signs and symptoms of a particular untold condition, who got progressively worse as time went on and would usually go into cardiac arrest – an absence of breathing and a pulse – which would be the worst case scenario in real life too, obviously! All the other candidates would be watching, staring at you, waiting for you to make a mistake; a mistake that, if it was a real patient, might have just made their condition worse or even killed them. Fortunately, the patient was just a mannequin – for now anyway – but a life-like mannequin that could be cannulated and intubated like a real person.

At the end of particular scenarios, which would sometimes have lasted thirty minutes to an hour to imitate a realistic period of time you might have a patient in your care – a patient whose life was in your hands – again with all the other candidates watching, Mr X would sternly question the treatment I had undertaken. We would sometimes end up in a heated debate over the treatment I had given to my fictitious patient. I would stand my ground though, especially when what I had done wasn't necessarily wrong or detrimental to the patient; I'd simply deviated a little from the JRCALC guidelines – a paramedic's bible – for the benefit of my patient. That's not forbidden as long as you can justify your actions; they're called guidelines as opposed to protocols for that very reason. However, you really do have to be able to justify your actions, or you could find yourself answering to the coroner.

Mr X and I would debate over whether I could justify my actions or not. However, our clash of personalities would eventually be addressed. I was called into his office for my end of week evaluation report, and he gave his opinion of me. He said,

'Andy, you're too argumentative.'

'No I'm not!' I abruptly replied. Umm... maybe he was right.

Nevertheless, and regardless of the fact that we may not have always got on like a house on fire, at the end of the twelve week course Mr X presented me with a 'Professional Paramedic Development Award' for most improved candidate. The course was over. I had done it; I had finally accomplished my ambition. And I had also taken the final step of my 'thousand mile journey' from postman to paramedic. It had taken me the best part of five years to achieve, but it was all worth it. And for my endeavours, I had received a prestigious award too. However, I was under no illusion that I'd learnt everything I ever needed to know on the course to be a proficient and professional paramedic. On the contrary, I was well aware that learning to be a professional paramedic had only just begun.

I will never forget that course for as long as I live; the instructors and the other course candidates were absolutely fantastic. And regardless of the fact that our personalities clashed, I will always have the utmost respect for Mr X for the rest of my life. His passion for the job was inspirational, his medical knowledge was exceptional, and his method of bringing out the best in people bordered on unbearable! Nevertheless, the hell he put me through on that course, without a doubt, not only prepared me for my impending *Baptism of Fire*, but would also prepare me for what I was going to endure as a professional paramedic for the rest of my NHS Ambulance Service career.

The Dark Side

Chapter 3
Hindsight

You often hear people say that police, fire and ambulance personnel become hardened to what they see and experience on a day-to-day basis, and I have to say there's a very small amount of truth in that statement – although I believe 'hardened' is the wrong word to use. Emergency service personnel do not necessarily become hardened to what they see, they simply accept that what they're exposed to is part of the job – adult or child, it goes with the territory. However, we are after all only human and therefore have emotions too.

A career in the Emergency Ambulance Service would not and does not suit everyone. I say 'does not' because I remember the story of a fellow employee several years ago. I didn't know him personally and I never met him, but the story travelled across the whole service at light speed. A young employee had successfully transferred from PTS to The Dark Side, full of enthusiasm and career ambition, and upon completing his technician training began his twelve month probationary period. On the very first day as part of a frontline ambulance crew, he attended to a fatal road traffic collision that involved two very young children. Understandably, that single, very sad and tragic incident was too much for him to bear. Needless to say, he quit immediately and returned to PTS duties.

You would think that the training syllabus would include footage or pictures of dead people, including children – to test the water, as it were – but no, it doesn't. It's a case of let's spend the money training you, and we'll see if you can hack it. Crazy!

Regardless of the fact that death is accepted as part of the job and that sad and tragic events are a normal part of everyday life, there are certain incidents paramedics attend to that can leave them feeling responsible for a patient's death. Not in a *Harold Shipman* type way, I hasten to add, more 'had their clinical decisions or actions have been different at the time, then the outcome may have been different' type of way. Fortunately, it is rare, but when it does happen then the only way to remove that feeling of 'I'm responsible' is to reflect on the incident and learn from it, and hope that you become a better health care professional as a consequence. Like I said, it rarely occurs, but nonetheless has happened to me, fortunately on one occasion only. I'll share that experience with you in considerable detail.

I was just three hours into a twelve hour day shift, crewed with Gemma, an ambulance technician. Gemma had a wacky, somewhat dizzy personality; she was great to work alongside, and shifts with her were usually full of laughter, but not always!

We were driving back to our base station one gloomy, overcast morning, hoping to get back for a cuppa, when to our disappointment the cab radio sounded. It was ambulance control dispatching us to a middle-aged female who was experiencing difficulty in breathing. Difficulty in breathing can be a sign and symptom of a myriad of medical conditions, but that's the only information we received. And that's the norm, as an ambulance crew is usually dispatched while the ambulance control room call-taker is still ascertaining information from the treble-nine caller. So Gemma activated the blue lights and sirens and put her foot down. She drove the six or seven miles to the given location and we had a bit of a giggle along the way; not at the forthcoming patient's expense, I hasten to add.

When we arrived at the address, which was a large, beautiful house on an affluent estate, Gemma and I hastily walked up the long paving-stoned driveway with the appropriate equipment in our possession.

'Hello... ambulance service!' I shouted through the front door that was ajar for our anticipated arrival.

'Up here,' a male voice replied from upstairs. We walked up the stairs, lugging all the equipment, and entered the bedroom, which was surprisingly small given the size of the house, but nonetheless beautifully decorated and furnished. We were met by a man standing over the bed trying to calm his wife, who the treble-nine had been dialled for. She was lying down, agitated and rolling around the bed, breathing rapidly, and was almost completely covered with an uber white duvet; only her feet and a small area of the calves of her legs were visible.

'Are her legs always that pale?' I asked the gent I correctly assumed was her husband, before introducing myself or even asking him what his concerns were.

'Yeah,' he calmly replied.

'OK... sorry, the colour of them took me by surprise then. Anyway, I'm Andy, this is Gemma. What's your wife's name, sir?'

'Margaret.'

'Hello Margaret, my name's Andy, I'm a paramedic. Can you slow your breathing down? You're breathing too fast, you sound like you're having a panic attack. Can you take the duvet off your face and sit up for me, please?' I calmly and politely asked.

'I'm gonna die! I'm gonna die!' she yelled from under the duvet in a way I'd heard before during incidents I'd attended on numerous occasions, where the patient was having a panic attack.

Panic attacks – or hyperventilating, to be more precise – are one of the many run-of-the-mill emergencies frontline ambulance staff attend to. The root cause of a panic attack usually occurs from a personal and/or psychological source. For example stress, which can obviously be caused by an abundance of reasons such as financial worries, relationship problems or fear of an upcoming event, such as an exam or job interview, to name but a few. The usual side effects of a panic attack are pins and needles down the arms and hands; also chest tightness, palpitations, and what is known as carpo-pedal spasm. This is when the wrist, and sometimes the feet, flexes and the fingers or toes gradually point inwards towards the body. All of the above mentioned side effects are caused by exhaling too much of the respiratory gas – carbon dioxide – due to rapid, shallow breathing. However, hyperventilating can also be caused by a serious underlying medical condition and not just anxiety alone.

'What's Margaret's history, sir?' I curiously asked her husband.

'Well, she's just been diagnosed with cervical cancer. She starts chemotherapy this Wednesday, and I think she's got herself all worked up over it. I think she's panicking because she's worried that if you take her into hospital then she's going to miss her chemotherapy appointment.'

'Oh, right. Well don't worry Margaret. If we need to take you into hospital and you're admitted, then a PTS ambulance will take you for your chemotherapy treatment on Wednesday, and bring you back, too. There's nothing to worry about, honestly,' I reassuringly explained to her, but still unable to see her face.

'I'm gonna die! I'm gonna die!' she exclaimed once again with sheer angst.

'Margaret, you're not going to die, just sit up for us please, calm down, and talk to us and let us help you,' I said, with reassurance. She blatantly ignored my request. I looked at Gemma with a discerning mono-brow.

'Can you talk to her, Gem? Try and coach her breathing,' I asked. Gemma leant over Margaret's bed.

'Margaret, slow your breathing down. Come on, honey. Can you take the duvet off your face and talk to us please?'

'I can't, I'm gonna die! I'm gonna die!' she said, yet again with a panic-stricken tone in her voice.

Margaret continued hyperventilating, with the duvet still covering her face and the majority of her body. We were doing our utmost best to reassure and reason with her. I felt helpless because my usual charming approach, which had worked on so many occasions in the past during other patient encounters, had absolutely no effect whatsoever. Gemma looked at me with a facial expression that asked 'what now?' However, I couldn't help but focus on Margaret's feet and calves.

'Her legs are very pale, chief. Are you sure they're always that pale?' I asked, frowning.

'Yeah, that's normal for her,' he calmly answered. With Margaret still in a state of incompliance, I looked at the ruffled duvet and gazed at her calves again, gradually becoming more and more concerned. A gut feeling was beginning to stir in my stomach.

'Right Margaret, you're going to have to sit up for us, my love. Lying face down under the duvet is not helping you to calm your breathing. So come on, sit up so we can help you. Come on!' I informed her with some assertion.

'I can't, I'm gonna die! I'm gonna die!' I took a deep breath and exhaled slowly.

'OK... Is she decent underneath the duvet, chief?'

'No... well, she's got her knickers on, but don't worry, just do what you have to do.'

'OK Gemma, let's pull the duvet back a bit, preserve her dignity as much as possible, and see if Margaret will sit up.' So I grabbed the scruff of the duvet at the head end and pulled it back slightly. Gemma and I immediately noticed how pale Margaret's face appeared, and it momentarily stunned us both. I'd never seen anyone so ghostly white in my life. Still shocked by the deathly appearance of her, I continued to encourage Margaret to comply with my request.

After several repeated attempts, Margaret finally complied with me and sat herself upright, with a little assistance from us. Her near-naked body was by now visible for the first time since we arrived at her bedside fifteen minutes or so ago, and she was whiter than white, as if she'd been rolled in a sack of flour. Gemma and I looked at each other with utter disbelief. Something wasn't right and we both knew it. And I don't think that the colour of her calves, that I'd been focusing on all along, was normal for her either, regardless of what her husband had said. She'd been hiding under the duvet all this time, her breathing going ten to the dozen and screaming at us that she was going to die; I was now beginning to believe that she had been right all along.

Sat up on the edge of the bed, Margaret stared into my eyes, not saying a word, not making a sound. Her breathing had almost instantaneously slowed down to that below a normal resting respiratory rate. The hyperventilating had suddenly stopped, which was unusual for somebody having a panic attack, as it usually slows gradually over several minutes or more, with encouragement, reassurance and coaching. She just sat there as white as snow, slouched with her head listing to one side, staring at me like she was possessed.

My heart began thumping against my chest because my adrenal glands had been suddenly awakened by the death-like appearance of her, and to the initially unforeseen, but now inevitable cardiac arrest that was about to ensue. Gemma and I leant over, looking directly at her face. Both of us were calling her name to get her attention, while staring into her eyes, when suddenly she had this brief episode of what I can only describe as a hypoxic fit, caused by an insufficient amount of oxygen reaching the brain. Then both of her pupils 'blew', that is, they went from reactive to changes in light, to fixed, non-reactive and dilated, within a millisecond, right before our very own eyes; a sure sign of sudden death. *Shit!* I thought, being very careful not to think aloud. Gemma looked at me, astonished and helpless.

'Get her on the floor quickly,' I abruptly said. While we quickly but carefully moved Margaret from the edge of the bed and on to the bedroom floor with accelerated haste, her husband understandably became concerned.

'Oh God, what's happening?' he asked.

'She's arrested, please leave the room sir, this isn't pleasant for you to watch. We'll do our best for her though, I assure you. Please leave now!' I said with an adrenal-fuelled dry mouth and tremor in my voice. Margaret's husband left the room, obviously concerned, confused, and with his head in his hands. 'Gem, apply the defibrillator pads; I'll start CPR.'

I commenced compressing her chest fifteen times in order for blood to be pumped around her body. I then pulled the BVM (bag and valve mask, which is used to ventilate a patient as an alternative to mouth-to-mouth), from the paramedic bag and attached it to the oxygen cylinder, and started ventilating Margaret. Within seconds, Gemma had applied the defibrillator pads and switched the machine on, and sadly the screen displayed asystole – that's a 'flatline' to the layperson. That means there is no electrical activity in the heart, no 'pumping' occurring, and therefore appears as a flat line on the ECG monitor; although, strictly speaking, it is not a perfect straight line. So Margaret's heart had suddenly ceased beating, and I couldn't understand why. She had been hyperventilating a minute ago and was now... dead.

Now, before I continue, I feel obliged to explain a few facts about defibrillation, as many lay-people assume – because of television programmes like *Casualty* and *Holby City* – that paramedics, nurses and doctors simply shock – or defibrillate, to be precise – patients back to life when they go into cardiac arrest. I wish it were that simple, but let me tell you now, it's not.

Firstly, not every patient who suffers a cardiac arrest is 'shockable', as it were. A patient's heart rhythm has to be displaying one of two specific rhythms on an ECG monitor in order for defibrillation to be an appropriate form of medical intervention. And even when the heart is in one of the two 'shockable' rhythms, unless the shock is applied within seconds of the cardiac arrest occurring, it is still seldom successful at restoring the heart to a rhythm compatible with life; although I'm glad to say it does happen, more so in the hospital environment where a doctor is available to apply immediate defibrillation. On the other hand, pre-hospital defibrillation is not so successful, unless there is a community defibrillator and trained personnel close-by. Why? Because it is more common for patients to collapse in cardiac arrest in the street or at home, and consequently, for each minute the heart goes without defibrillation, the chance of restoring the heart to a rhythm compatible with life diminishes.

In Margaret's case, defibrillation was not an appropriate form of treatment, because her heart rhythm was in neither of the two 'shockable' rhythms. However, the clinician can still view a patient's post cardiac arrest heart rhythm using the defibrillator pads; that is common practice, as it saves precious time not having to attach an ECG lead to each individual limb of a patient's body. Anyway, now I've cleared that up, let's continue with the story.

'Gemma, get that sewing stool and elevate her legs,' I indicated, 'it'll encourage her blood pressure, and then take over chest compressions while I try and intubate 'er.' Gemma moved the stool and raised Margaret's legs, then commenced chest compressions as I had instructed. Margaret's eyes were still wide open, and for some reason it never once occurred to me to brush my hand over her eyelids to close them while we tried to resuscitate her. I continued ventilating, while I simultaneously prepared the intubation equipment.

Between ventilations, I used the one free hand I had to push the bed out of the way, to increase the amount of space available for me to attempt intubation; the other hand was securing the ventilating mask over Margaret's face. During training in the hospital theatres, the patient was on an operating table four feet off the ground, with ample space for us to manoeuvre. In the pre-hospital environment, the patient is obviously in no position to consider, when they collapse and die, how much space is needed for a paramedic to work, or more importantly, intubate.

I informed Gemma that I was ready to attempt intubation, so I asked her to stop compressions so the movement of the body didn't obscure my view of the vocal chords. I held the laryngoscope – used to shift the tongue to the left – in my left hand, with an appropriately sized tube in my right. Then I held my breath and placed the laryngoscope into Margaret's mouth and moved her tongue over to the left, and attempted to view Margaret's vocal chords.

The reason I held my own breath was because, during training, it was emphasised that if you, the clinician, felt the need to breathe yourself, then you should cease your attempt at intubation and ventilate the patient for a short time before another go at securing a tube is attempted. In this way, the patient does not go un-oxygenated or un-ventilated for a prolonged period of time, as intubating can be very problematic on those patients with particularly difficult anatomical airways.

Fortunately, Margaret's airway was classed as a 'Grade One' of four grades of difficulty. Therefore, I inserted the tube with relative ease and secured it in place, before placing my stethoscope over various positions of her chest to listen to her lung fields while squeezing the ventilating bag attached to the end of the tube, to ensure correct placement. I instructed Gemma to continue with compressions. At the same time, I attached the automatic ventilator to the end of the tube, leaving my hands free to gain IV access.

As I moved myself away from the head end of Margaret and towards the side of her, I noticed her stomach appeared somewhat 'rotund'.

'Gemma, do you think 'er stomach seems unusually big for the size of her frame?' I asked, with a confused expression.

'Yeah... what you thinking?' she asked while panting away, performing chest compressions.

'Umm... I definitely saw the tube pass through the vocal chords, and I listened to 'er lung fields. There's no way I went into the oesophagus.' That's the 'food pipe' to the layperson. If I had inserted the tube into the oesophagus, then every time the automatic ventilator forced air into her, the air would be entering her stomach as opposed to her lungs. That would be frowned upon by a doctor or a coroner if it hadn't been recognised by the paramedic, or it was recognised but the paramedic did nothing to remedy the problem – that is, withdraw the tube and try again. 'No... the tube is definitely where it should be, I'm positive.' I pondered for a moment. 'No, there's something else... there's another reason. I'm thinking a bleed... a *triple A* maybe.'

A 'triple A' (AAA) is an abbreviation for 'Abdominal Aortic Aneurism'. The aorta is the largest artery in the human body. If it suddenly ruptures then the prognosis is extremely poor without rapid surgical intervention. The patient literally bleeds to death internally, and as a consequence, the stomach tends to swell very quickly from the litres of blood accumulating.

'OK, keep going Gemma, I'll get a cannula in and put a bag of fluid up and push some drugs through.' I unclipped the tourniquet from around my trouser belt and positioned it around Margaret's arm, and pulled it tight in order to cause blood to engorge her by now collapsing veins. From the paramedic bag, I chose a large bore cannula used for rapid fluid administration, which is what my plan was. I needed to get some fluid into Margaret to replace the blood she had potentially lost, if my diagnosis of a 'triple A' was correct. However, Margaret was by now extremely shut down. The tourniquet was having an undesired effect, and her veins were only just viable for cannulation thanks to the skill and success of the compressions Gemma was doing, forcing the veins to engorge due to the effect of the blood being 'pushed' around the body.

I prepared the area of Margaret's arm I was intending to cannulate, and then removed the long, wide cannula from its packaging. My hands were shaking from the ongoing effects of adrenaline caused by the sudden change in Margaret's life-status. I patted her arm where the vein was and pierced the skin with the needle. The flashback appeared in the chamber. I advanced the needle further. The secondary flashback appeared along the length of the clear plastic tube. I unclipped the tourniquet, applied digital pressure to the vein and withdrew the needle, and discarded the needle into the sharps container. I screwed the Luer-Lock to the end and quickly secured it in place with an adhesive dressing, before flushing it with a ten-millilitre pre-filled syringe of sodium chloride to confirm patent IV access.

'OK, let's get some drugs into her,' I said, thinking out aloud while unzipping the drugs bag. I pulled out a pre-filled syringe of adrenaline, cracked it open, removed the caps, screwed the male and female parts together and pushed the contents through the cannula situated in Margaret's vein. Adrenaline is administered to patients in cardiac arrest because it is classed as a vasoconstrictor, which, to keep it simple, narrows the blood vessels and encourages an increase in blood pressure and cardiac output – that is, the volume of blood being pumped by the heart.

I then opened a pre-filled syringe of atropine, removed the caps, screwed the two pieces together and pushed the contents of that syringe through the cannula too. Atropine contains an extract from the deadly nightshade plant. Its effect, when given intravenously, encourages an increase in heart rate; although at the time of writing this book, atropine has since been removed from the UK resuscitation guidelines.

'Gemma, stop compressions. I'll take over, you have a rest. Set me up a bag of sodium chloride though, will ya.' I took over the compressions and Gemma hurriedly prepared a bag of fluid for me. While I was performing compressions, I began to think about the next stage of my plan. I had to decide whether to move Margaret to the ambulance and rush her to hospital, continuing with CPR, or continue CPR in the bedroom – 'load and go' or 'stay and play', as we call it in the ambulance service. The only reservation I had was that moving her on to an ambulance carry chair and descending the stairs would mean temporarily ceasing resuscitation.

Statistically, successful resuscitation from a 'flatline' rhythm is one percent. If I were to temporarily cease resuscitation to move Margaret, then the chances of reviving her were minimal; and historically, if ambulance personnel arrive at A&E with a patient in a 'flatline' rhythm, the doctors tend to confirm death within seconds or minutes of their arrival anyway.

So after some careful consideration, I made the decision to continue on scene and give her the benefit of the doubt of uninterrupted resuscitation for a while longer. It was a tough decision, but the right one as far as I was concerned. Gemma had by now prepared the fluid, so she recommenced chest compressions and I quickly attached the giving set to the cannula in Margaret's arm, hung it up on the bedroom radiator and let the contents run freely.

Margaret was being automatically ventilated; Gemma was performing continuous chest compressions; I'd administered an initial dose of adrenaline and the one and only required dose of atropine. There was a bag of IV fluid in situ, set to run rapidly, and her feet were elevated. There was nothing else Gemma and I could do, other than to continue with CPR and administer adrenaline every three minutes until Margaret responded or her heart rhythm converted to a 'shockable' rhythm; defibrillation would then be indicated and an additional drug would have been administered, once only, in addition to adrenaline.

We continued Advanced Cardiac Life Support measures for a further twenty minutes, with no change in ECG rhythm compatible with life. There were no clinical signs that Margaret was breathing for herself; no evidence of a return of spontaneous circulation – that is, a pulse – and her pupils remained fixed and dilated. Sadly, Margaret was not responding to CPR, drug and fluid therapy. She was dead. We had to accept that she was gone and no amount of CPR was going to bring her back. So Gemma and I both agreed that resuscitation should be ceased. I switched the ventilator off and clamped the fluid so it was no longer running, and Gemma stopped performing chest compressions.

I came to my feet from the kneeling position I had adopted throughout the entire resuscitation attempt. With my legs now seized up, I rubbed my forehead in disbelief of how this call had started out, but how it had now ended. I couldn't believe it. I'd actually said to Margaret, 'You're not going to die.' I'd reassured her; I'd given her my word. I felt like I'd let her down, and let her husband down too. Now I had to go and break the news to him. What was I going to say? I'd broken bad news to deceased patients' loved ones numerous times, but this was different. He'd heard me say to her that she wasn't going to die.

I took another look at Margaret lying dead on the carpeted bedroom floor, and began to prepare myself to go and tell her husband the unexpected news.

'I hate this bit,' I thought, as I vacated the bedroom and wandered around the upstairs of the house looking for him. He heard my footsteps and appeared from another bedroom. I took a deep breath and then tactfully explained to him that Margaret had died, and although we had done our utmost best to resuscitate her for over twenty minutes, she had not responded to treatment. Obviously distraught, he put his head into his hands and sobbed his heart out. I asked him if there was anything I could do to help him at such a difficult time, like contact a family member or a close neighbour. While still crying in disbelief, he informed me that he would do that.

I went back into the bedroom where Gemma was and asked her to put the duvet over Margaret's body. We had no choice but to leave the tube and cannula, with fluid attached, in place for post-mortem purposes, which was the procedure following a pre-hospital cardiac arrest. Gemma then went to the ambulance to get the paperwork for me to complete, while I re-joined Margaret's husband and directed him towards an armchair.

I explained to him that I didn't know what had happened to Margaret, but that I thought she may have had a spontaneous internal bleed; however, a post-mortem would confirm her cause of death. I also explained to him that the police would be contacted, not because there was anything suspicious about what had happened, but because the police act on behalf of the Coroner's Office. He understood, but was obviously still very shocked.

When Gemma returned with the paperwork, I sat and completed the appropriate forms while waiting for the police to arrive. They took me a little while to complete because of all the events leading up to Margaret being pronounced dead, including the invasive treatment and interventions Gemma and I had carried out during the incident; all had to be carefully and accurately documented. Interestingly, there's a saying in the medical profession, 'If you didn't document it, you didn't do it'.

I also had to complete a Recognition of Life Extinct, or ROLE form, as paramedics – although not able to certify a patient's death

– are able to recognise that a patient is no longer living, prior to or following resuscitation attempts. Excluding particular circumstances and patient presentations, a paramedic can choose not to begin resuscitation, or continue with resuscitation if bystander CPR has been commenced, if they feel that the patient's presentations are not compatible with life. For instance, if a patient is rigor mortised – that is, has post death stiffening of the body – and has evidently been deceased for some considerable time.

When the police arrived, I explained the unfortunate, sad and tragic circumstances and directed them to the bedroom where Margaret lay, and upon the police being satisfied that there were no suspicious circumstances, Gemma and I paid our respects to Margaret's husband and then vacated the house. We placed the equipment back into the saloon of the ambulance and informed Control that we were now clear and available for a further call. Fortunately, the remainder of the shift was relatively quiet, and we were only dispatched to straightforward calls that didn't involve anything sombre; although throughout the remainder of the shift, I couldn't get Margaret out of my mind.

Later that night, while at home with my wife and children, I was unusually quiet. I couldn't help but think about Margaret and the fear she must have been feeling while rolling around, agitated, under the duvet. I thought about her husband and how he was coping that evening without his wife. I'd seen pictures of their daughters hung up on the living room walls and displayed on cabinets. How had they taken the sudden loss of their mum? I also thought about how I'd seen hundreds of dead people since joining the ambulance service but not once felt the way I did then – guilty and responsible. I could only assume it was because all of the other dead people I'd seen were dead before I arrived at their side. The circumstances surrounding Margaret's death were somewhat more difficult to comprehend, because she was alive when Gemma and I had arrived to help her, and then, less than an hour later, I confirmed her dead.

Several weeks went by and, while on a day shift, I bumped into Gemma at the ambulance station.

'Remember Margaret we went to a few weeks ago?'

'Of course,' I thought, 'how could I possibly forget that incident!' but answered 'Yeah, why do you ask?'

'Well, I did a job,' she said, meaning an emergency call, 'on the same estate the other day, a friend of Margaret's. They told me that the post-mortem revealed that she died of an aortic aneurism,' Gemma added informatively.

That didn't surprise me whatsoever. I was almost certain it was a 'triple A' within the first ten minutes of resuscitating her; her deathly pallor and swollen stomach gave it away. The cogs began turning again. What if I had pulled the duvet completely off when we arrived, and acted on the suspicious pale colour of her calves, instead of allowing her to lie beneath the duvet for so long? I would have put two and two together. What if I had requested another crew and removed her to the ambulance horizontally on a scoop stretcher? That would've been very difficult to do throughout the entire extraction from the bedroom, but it may have kept her blood pressure at a sufficient level, and kept her alive long enough for a surgeon to open her up, find the location of the aortic rupture and save her life. It's obviously a lot more complex and sophisticated than that, but what if?

What if? What if? What if? Hindsight, it's the perfect science, isn't it!

I pondered over that incident for several weeks, reflecting on my actions, asking myself repeatedly whether she would have survived had I kept her horizontal throughout – or asked her to lie back down, or assisted her to lie back down, after she had sat up on the edge of the bed. I will never know. But to dwell on hindsight will destroy you, whether you're a paramedic or not. So instead, I chose to learn from that experience and hoped I would become a better paramedic as a consequence.

I'll never forget that incident; unfortunately, it will stay with me for the rest of my life. And although Margaret was the first patient to be living one minute and then dead the next while still in my presence, unfortunately and unbeknown to me at the time, she wouldn't be the last.

The Dark Side

Chapter 4
Shutdown

One of the most interesting aspects of being a paramedic is not knowing what you're going to attend to next. It's so unpredictable. You could be parked up at some stand-by point discussing the football, relationships or what you intend to do during your days off, or have your feet up in the ambulance station watching TV. You may have just dealt with a run-of-the-mill teenager having an anxiety attack, or a motorist who's had a minor rear-end shunt on the carriageway – easy dealings, you know. But then your body is rudely awakened by the sudden side effects of adrenaline when the radio alarms and you're dispatched to a life-threatening emergency. You go from being slouched in an armchair in the ambulance station or the front seat of an ambulance, feeling tired and lethargic, with a horizontal-like attitude to life, to a sudden change in posture: alert, ready for action, and ready to put your skills and knowledge at the forefront of your mind. Your thinking cap is on; your clinical thought processes are poised, ready to act on your arrival at the patient's side.

Well, it's like that at first anyway, during a day in the life of a paramedic. But after a while, when you've experienced it hundreds, maybe thousands of times, and have the self-confidence in your ability to handle most circumstances that are thrown at you, and become almost completely desensitised to adrenal-fuelled action, then it takes a particular incident to bring that adrenaline rush back into play; for example, a life-threatening paediatric emergency, motorcyclist versus car, or a pedestrian versus bus. I've attended a few of them. Now *they* can make you twitch a bit, because you don't know what you are going to find on your arrival at the scene. The patient tends to be either dead, traumatically injured but 'viable', or rubbing a 'hurty' knee, shoulder or head... because it wasn't strictly a 'pedestrian versus bus', the patient merely stepped off the curb while the bus was moving off from a bus stop.

An even better example is a minibus crash with school children on board. Now that gets the adrenaline going, I assure you! The anticipation of not knowing how many children are involved, or what state you will find them in on your arrival, causes an adrenal release like no other. Actually, while I'm on the subject of minibuses, children and adrenaline, I'll have to tell you a little humorous story about a few former colleagues of mine. I'll call them Brian, Pete and Del.

Brian was a veteran paramedic, and a very good one, too. But he was renowned for being a bit stressy and impatient, a bit of a 'flapper', you know the type. Consequently, he was often the victim of banter. Brian was working a night shift crewed with Del, another paramedic. At about 3 a.m., while Brian and Del were parked up under the canopy of the A&E ambulance bay, Pete arrived with a patient in his ambulance. After Pete had handed his patient over to the A&E staff, he began chatting to Del in private, away from Brian who was still sat in the cab of the ambulance, dozing off.

Following their brief conversation, Del adopted his position back in the attendant's seat of the ambulance. While Pete was stood talking to Del through the wound down passenger door window, they both began making conversation with Brian, who was intermittently nodding off. Del then turned to Brian, whose eyes were closed, and said,

'Blimey Brian, imagine gettin' called to a minibus crash now on the motorway, full of children, it'd be bloody awful wouldn't it, 'cause you're knackered aren't ya?'

'It doesn't bear thinkin' about, mate,' Brian replied, with his eyes closed, arms crossed and chin on his chest.

Moments later the cab radio sounded, so Brian, startled, answered it,

'Go ahead, over.'

'Roger, RED call to a sixteen-seat minibus RTC, M-fifty-six northbound. Approximately eight children on board but exact number of casualties unknown yet, over,' the male voice said over the radio, with a sense of urgency in his voice.

'Jesus Christ! What are the chances of that?!' Brian asked, shocked at the coincidence. He immediately went into a flapping frenzy, rocking back and forth in his seat, breathing rapidly, and at the same time repeatedly slapped the back of his own head from sheer anxiety and anticipation of such a potentially stressful looming emergency call. Del and Pete burst into laughter and nearly pissed themselves watching Brian panic and damn near soil his uniform.

It turned out that Del and Pete had contacted their mate in the ambulance control centre and asked him to pass Brian the fictitious motorway emergency on their signal, which was to be a text message to say that they had laid the bait, now quickly pass the coincidental call. The prank went like clockwork, and the story travelled from crew-to-crew throughout the remainder of the shift. Brilliant! A sick sense of humour you may think, but they're the sort of pranks that occur in the ambulance service. And believe me, I could tell you a lot more stories about pranks that have been pulled, by me on others, from others on me, and from others on other personnel. It's part of the job, and part of the fantastic camaraderie of being in the ambulance service.

Anyway, like I said, it takes a particular incident to bring that adrenaline rush back into play. But there is often no warning; you can be caught off guard. What might seem like a routine, run-of-the-mill call after the details are passed to you via the radio, can actually turn out to be one of those adrenal-fuelled encounters. It is common for an ambulance crew to be given very little information about their forthcoming patient's condition. You might receive information such as 'sixty year-old female with shortness of breath' or 'seventy year-old male with chest pain' and that's it. Both of them can be something or nothing.

So when Gemma and I were dispatched to a fifty-two year-old male, diabetic unresponsive, my adrenal glands remained asleep for the duration of the seven minute blue-light drive to the address given, because the first thing that went through my mind was a straightforward unresponsive diabetic who had low blood sugar levels. When I say straightforward, I mean you turn up, pop a cannula in the arm, infuse some glucose and bring them back around; then carry out some vital observations. Job done. But, like I said, you can be caught off guard – as this next incident I attended to emphasises exactly.

It was 9:30 a.m. on a cold winter's morning, and Gemma and I were parked up on stand-by. We had already attended to two very poorly patients, for whom I had requested resus due to their life-threatening presentations. We both got the impression it was going to be one of those days, where you start as you mean to go on. At 9:45 a.m., still parked up, the cab radio sounded.

'Go ahead, over.'

'Roger, RED call to a fifty-two year-old male, diabetic unresponsive, over,' the dispatcher said.

'Roger that, over.' So Gemma activated the blue lights and sirens and drove to the address given, which was on a poverty-stricken council estate renowned for drug and alcohol abuse. When we arrived on the doorstep, with equipment in our possession, we were met by the patient's wife, who directed us to the outside of a locked, upstairs bathroom. I placed the equipment on the floor and turned to the concerned lady,

'What's the problem, my love?' I politely asked.

'Well, he took the dog for a walk this morning about eight-thirty, and when he came back, about nine-thirty, he said he felt unwell and was shaking. So he went straight to the bathroom but he's been in there about twenty, twenty-five minutes, and he's not come out. I've been calling his name for the last ten minutes, before and since calling for an ambulance, but he's not responding. I'm concerned 'cause he's diabetic,' she explained.

'Yeah, the controller said. Is he type one or two?' I asked.

'Type one. He uses insulin.'

'OK, what's his name, love?'

'Jim.' So I knocked on the bathroom door.

'Jim! Jim! Can you hear me? It's the paramedics,' I shouted. I waited silently, with my ear to the door. There was no response. 'Jim! Can you hear me? It's the paramedics,' I repeated. There was still no response. 'I might 'ave to kick the bathroom door in hun, I'm sorry.'

'No, that's OK.'

'Right, step back a bit,' I advised Gemma and Jim's wife. I crouched down on the floor and peeked under the small gap underneath the door, to make sure that Jim was not immediately behind it. There was light, so I assumed the door was safe to break in without causing any injury to him. I kicked at the door with the sole of my boot. BANG! No joy. BANG! No joy. BANG! Still no joy. 'Bloody 'ell, where are we, Fort Knox?' I thought. BANG! The door flew open. I was expecting to find Jim stationary and unconscious. But when I entered the bathroom, which was tiny and would not have fitted more than myself and him in, he was having a severe seizure – no doubt but not yet confirmed – caused by a diabetic hypoglycaemic episode.

Before I continue, let me explain a little about diabetes. Diabetes is a condition that involves the failure of the pancreas to produce insulin (type-1), or an inadequate ability to produce insulin (type-2). Type-1 is generally diagnosed as a child, and type-2 – more commonly known as 'late onset diabetes' – is generally caused by obesity; although people with type-2 sometimes progress to type-1. If a diabetic patient does not control their condition adequately or responsibly, they can experience low blood sugar levels, or hypoglycaemia, to be precise – more commonly known in the medical profession as a 'hypo'. Conversely, a paramedic might also attend to a patient with high blood sugar levels, a condition better known as hyperglycaemia. Either of them can be fatal if not treated in a timely manner.

Jim was a big guy. He was wedged between the toilet and the bath in a position that no human could possibly tolerate if conscious. He was evidently convulsing. His entire body was rigid and his mouth was jammed shut, a side effect of convulsing and many other conditions, known as trismus. Seizures often cause the patient to bite their tongue due to trismus, which makes it impossible to insert an oral airway adjunct.

I wanted to move him from the awkward position he was in, but because he was wedged it proved impossible, especially while he was convulsing. I confirmed his AVPU as U – unresponsive – and his GCS as three, out of a possible fifteen. I leant over, precariously stepping over and around his convulsing body, with no choice but to adopt a very uncomfortable position to avoid standing on him. I was practically playing *Twister* in his bathroom. Gemma then passed me a lubricated nasopharyngeal airway, so I inserted it with a twisting motion into his right nostril, to ensure a patent airway. She then passed me the oxygen cylinder with a mask attached, so I placed the mask over his face and administered high flow oxygen to him.

With an airway secured and breathing confirmed, I felt for a pulse in his wrist. He had one. It was weak, but he had one. The colour and feel of him took me a little by surprise. He was grey, cold to the touch and very clammy, so there was no point in placing the sats probe on him, as it rarely measures accurate saturations of oxygen when placed on a cold, clammy finger.

Remaining in an awkward position, I restrained his hand, with some difficulty due to him convulsing, and then cleaned the index finger of his right hand with some gauze soaked in tap water, to ensure that nothing sugary was on his finger, as that would cause an inaccurate blood sugar measurement. I prepared the glucometer and then, once again, restrained his hand and pin-pricked his index finger for a drop of blood, carefully placing the small amount that oozed from the minute wound on to the measuring strip of the glucometer. While I waited for the digital measurement to display a figure, I ascertained some information from his wife who was stood outside of the bathroom, alongside Gemma, calm but evidently concerned.

'Right my love, he's diabetic, yeah? Has he eaten today?' I asked.

'No, he skipped breakfast this morning, but still injected his insulin, and then took the dog for a walk.'

'Is that normal for him to skip breakfast?'

'Er… no, it's not, not really.'

'Does he have any other history at all? I take it he's not a diagnosed epileptic as well as diabetic, is he?'

'No, he's not epileptic. But he's had two heart attacks and a heart bypass graft years ago.'

'Does he generally manage his diabetes well, would you say?'

'Not brilliantly, 'cause he drinks.'

'Oh, that's not good is it, alcohol when ya diabetic. When was his last hypo?'

'Er… I don't know. A few months ago, I think.'

'OK, cheers love.'

With some relevant information obtained from his wife, I glanced down at the glucometer. It displayed a decimalised blood glucose measurement of just nought point seven *millimoles per litre of blood*, which is usually written as 0.7mmol/l. That is dangerously low, and was probably lower than what was displayed on the glucometer, as they only measure an estimate; a very good estimate, but nonetheless an estimate.

Hypoglycaemia is considered as a blood sugar level below 4.0mmol/l. He was at serious risk of going into cardiac arrest if I didn't rapidly intervene, as the brain requires glucose to survive (to keep it simple). If the body's blood sugar falls too low, there is a risk of deterioration, and ultimately death.

Jim presented similarly to an elderly diabetic I attended to some time ago. He too had suffered a hypoglycaemic episode, and had convulsed as a consequence. On arrival of my crewmate and I at his side, he took his last breaths and went into cardiac arrest within a minute. And although advanced life support measures were performed for over twenty minutes, with glucose administered, he didn't respond to treatment and, sadly, I pronounced him dead at the scene.

Unconsciousness due to a diabetic hypoglycaemic episode varies from diabetic to diabetic. Some diabetics remain conscious and alert when their blood sugar levels are 2.0mmol/l, some are merely confused and slur their speech, and then others become unconscious. However, I've yet to attend to a patient who is still conscious with a blood sugar level below 1.0mmol/l, and I'm unlikely to either.

I quickly applied a tourniquet to his right arm, with a view to cannulating and administering intravenous glucose. I tapped his arm to try and get a vein to reveal itself, but no joy. He was so shutdown that cannulation access sites were poor in his right arm. So I left the tourniquet in place and applied another tourniquet to his left arm. After a minute or so of tapping over venous sites, there was, once again, no joy.

My lower back was absolutely killing from the awkward position I was in, trying to restrain Jim's arm while looking for an IV access site. My uncomfortable posture was causing beads of sweat to roll down my forehead. So I unclipped the tourniquet from around his left arm, so blood flow wasn't restricted for a prolonged period, and placed the right sided tourniquet further down, around his wrist, to gauge whether there was a vein in his hand.

'Can't you find a vein?' Gemma asked me from outside the bathroom, poised ready to setup a glucose drip on confirmation that I had IV access.

'No, he's completely shutdown. We might have to scoop and run,' I said, with adrenaline coursing through my veins. I took a couple of deep breaths and continued to tap Jim's right hand. I could have chanced an attempt at cannulating his arm where a vein should physiologically be, but as he was convulsing, that would likely prove unsuccessful. 'Come on. Come on, reveal yourself,' I muttered to myself while tapping. Nothing viable was appearing. 'Bloody 'ell,' I thought, 'this is not looking good.'

If I was presented with the same situation today, it would be a different scenario altogether, because paramedics have equipment that allows us to drill a needle into the bone of the leg or shoulder. It would still be difficult in a convulsing patient, but easier than the predicament I was in during this incident. Jim was a very, very poorly man. Death was imminent.

Convulsing isn't dissimilar to isometric exercise. Isometric exercises are a type of strength training in which the joint angle and muscle length do not change during contraction. Isometrics are done in static positions, rather than being dynamic through a range of motion, so Jim would be metabolising calories, or 'burning sugar', causing his blood sugar levels to drop too, to the point that he would stop convulsing and deteriorate into cardiac arrest within minutes.

The pressure was on and I could feel the effects of adrenaline trying to get the better of me, but I refused to begin panicking, regardless of the fact that if I didn't gain IV access very soon, he was going to die; and the distance to hospital was about ten miles. Plus, we would first have to extract him from the bathroom, down the stairs and into the ambulance while he was still convulsing, and rely on nothing but diesel for the journey to hospital. That plan would be an absolute logistical nightmare, let me tell you, and one neither I, nor Gemma were in favour of. In fact, carrying a convulsing patient down the stairs on a carry chair was fraught with danger for us all. One slip could retire us all!

With Jim still violently convulsing and a tourniquet around his wrist, I restrained his arm and began tapping his hand, hoping for a suitable vein to appear; just a small one would suffice, anything just to get some glucose into him. Paramedics do carry an oral drug called Hypostop, but to administer Hypostop, your patient has to have a gag-reflex and be able to swallow; so that was a non-starter, as Jim was unconscious.

Paramedics also carry a drug that is administered into the muscle, called Glucagon. Glucagon is made naturally in the pancreas; its purpose is to allow glycogen, in the form of glucose, to be secreted into the bloodstream when sugar levels are low. However, it is unlikely to work if the glycogen in the liver is extremely low, which Jim's more than likely was. His blood sugar was life-threateningly low and he had administered his insulin that morning, therefore the glycogen stores in his liver were more than likely to be depleted. However, if I couldn't gain IV access, I would have no choice but to administer Glucagon in the off-chance that it worked, and then scoop and run to the nearest A&E, ten miles away.

I could feel myself getting warmer and warmer, flushed and sweaty from the time-critical predicament and because of the extremely stressful posture I had to adopt while trying to gain IV access. Jim continued to violently convulse, while Gemma and his wife looked on. I don't think his wife understood the seriousness of the situation. I was glad too, because that can increase the pressure put on you as the paramedic, regardless of the fact that I'd learnt to remain calm on the outside even though my heart was pounding on the inside.

When you attend to a patient having a hypoglycaemic episode, the majority of the time their blood sugar levels are low, but not necessarily life-threateningly low. You have ample time to gain IV access (without difficulty) and administer glucose before they're anywhere close to death. Jim was only moments from death, and every second he was convulsing there was a greater chance that his blood sugar level would reduce further and further. With the tourniquet still in place around the wrist of his right hand, I continued tapping away, hoping that a vein of any size would appear, and a viable one at that. After a couple more minutes of quite hard tapping, a very small and narrow vein appeared under the pale, cold, clammy skin of his hand.

'I think I might 'ave one Gem, pass me a blue cannula, quick!'

Gemma quickly opened the packaged cannula and passed it to me. So, still restraining Jim's right arm, I carefully, with intense concentration and my legs and hands shaking from the stressful position I had no choice but to adopt, pierced the skin and entered the vein. A very modest flashback appeared in the chamber, so I advanced it further and awaited a secondary flashback along the length of the clear plastic tube. The secondary flashback appeared. I unclipped the tourniquet, applied digital pressure to the vein and withdrew the needle, and although not professional clinical practice, I had no choice but to temporarily throw the sharp needle into the sink, situated to my left, in order to keep hold of his wrist. I then screwed the Luer-Lock to the end.

While still restraining his arm as he continued to convulse, I couldn't help but think to myself, if I let go now, without the cannula secured, I'll lose the only opportunity I have of preventing him from going into cardiac arrest. With great difficulty, I scruffily applied an adhesive dressing over and around the cannula to secure it in place. Gemma then passed me a pre-filled syringe of sodium chloride to flush the cannula and confirm it was patent and accurately placed. As Jim was so clammy, and because the adhesive dressings come away easily on clammy skin, I protected the IV access further by wrapping a net-like bandage around it, which would make it more difficult to pull or knock it out, as patients who are convulsing often do.

With the cannula now secured and flushed, Gemma had pre-empted my plan to administer IV diabetic juice, so passed me a prepared bag of ten percent glucose. So, once again I restrained Jim's arm, unscrewed the Luer-Lock and attached the glucose giving set to the cannula. I asked Jim's wife to fetch me a coat hanger from the bedroom, so I could hang the drip up and allow the contents to run freely. Because I had no choice but to use the smallest cannula that paramedics carry, usually used for children, the only problem was it was going to take a few minutes for the 50 millilitres of glucose, which I intended to initially administer, to enter his circulation and ultimately increase his blood sugar levels.

The sweat was dripping down my forehead because I had been in such an awkward and uncomfortable position for several minutes, and because adrenaline was racing through my veins, believing that, from his presentation, he was minutes away from cardiac arrest – for the sake of a bit of 'sugar'!

The three of us waited patiently for the glucose to take effect, and as expected, slowly but surely Jim's convulsing began to slow down, until it stopped completely after approximately 50 millilitres of the glucose had entered his veins.

'Thank Christ for that', I thought. So I began my attempts at rousing him. 'Jim! Jim! Can you hear me? It's the ambulance service. Jim! Jim! Open your eyes for me,' I calmly requested. Jim opened his eyes and looked at me. He appeared confused, as diabetics often are when they initially rouse. 'Hello Jim. My name's Andy, I'm a paramedic. You've had a hypo, mate,' I informed him. He just stared at me, perplexed, with a look of fear in his eyes. He then began lashing out, throwing harmless, child-like punches while wedged between the toilet and the bath. He still tolerated the tube inserted into his right nostril and didn't even acknowledge that it was there. 'Calm down Jim, calm down. It's OK, you've had a hypo, mate,' I repeated.

After a couple of minutes, he moved himself from between the toilet and the bath, and shuffled in to a foetal position on the bathroom floor, closed his eyes and went unconscious again.

'That's odd,' I thought. So I took the opportunity to take another blood glucose measurement. That second test measured 5.5mmol/l. 'Excellent,' I thought, 'the glucose drip has been a success,' or at least I thought it had! A couple of minutes later, Jim spontaneously opened his eyes, saw me and began swearing at me and lashing out again. His combative behaviour concerned me, as his blood glucose reading of 5.5mmol/l did not reflect the conscious level and behaviour I was witnessing. Something was wrong!

Jim continued to thrash about, but eventually went unconscious once again. I didn't interfere with him; I just took the opportunity to administer a further 25 millilitres of glucose. Several minutes passed by, and Jim gradually began to wake. He looked at me, this time with less confusion, and didn't throw any haymakers in my direction.

'Hello Jim. Are you OK? You've had a hypo. Just relax though, mate, there's no rush,' I said, attempting to reassure him.

'What's 'appened?' he asked, pulling out the tube from his nostril, looking at it, confused as to what it was, before placing it onto the floor.

'You've had a hypo, love,' his wife uttered from outside the bathroom door.

'Can I just pin-prick your finger again and see what your sugar levels are at now?' I asked. He didn't answer; he just held a hand out for me. So, for the third time, I measured his blood glucose level, and to my alarm it was back down to 2.8mmol/l.

'I don't believe it, what the hell's going on?' I thought. I was very concerned. Something just didn't add up. 'We need to get Jim into the ambulance as quick as possible,' I said, alternating my eyes between Gemma and Jim's wife. 'At least then, if he deteriorates, he's in the ambulance and we can use diesel,' I said. Gemma went down the stairs and outside to fetch the carry chair from the ambulance, and to prepare the stretcher for Jim's imminent arrival.

On her return, Gemma placed the carry chair outside of the bathroom.

'Jim... Jim. Do you think you could stand to your feet and sit on our chair? It's just outside the bathroom, mate. We need to take you to hospital for further check-ups; your blood sugars aren't right. OK?' Jim understood my request, complied, slowly stood to his feet, walked out of the bathroom and sat on the carry chair. Gemma and I then carried him down the stairs, out of the front door, along the garden path, and into the back of the ambulance, accompanied by his wife, who was coming to hospital with us. So I offered her a seat and asked Jim to position himself on the stretcher, and ensured he was sat semi-recumbent, as my assessment of him was far from complete!

'Right, Gemma, get me a blood pressure, temperature and another blood glucose measurement will ya, hun. I'm gonna get the twelve lead ECG on.'

'OK mate,' she replied.

A 12 Lead ECG actually only consists of ten leads. Six leads are placed across the left side of the chest, and a lead is positioned on each limb. The term 12 Lead ECG derives from the fact that it analyses the rhythm of the heart from twelve different angles. 12 Lead ECGs are used to assist a paramedic diagnose various conditions. However, its primary purpose is to diagnose heart attacks.

I dried Jim's sweaty, clammy chest with paper towel, so I could apply the sticky, gel covered ECG electrodes to his chest. Then with him lying still, and the ECG prepared, I pressed the record button and waited the few seconds it takes for the monitor to analyse the rhythm of the patient's heart. The machine printed a rhythm strip. To my alarm, there was evidence to suggest that Jim may be having a heart attack.

The cause of high or low blood sugar levels in a diabetic can be due to a heart attack, often a silent heart attack. By 'silent' I mean the patient does not feel chest pain. It is common for diabetics to suffer a heart attack either with or without chest pain – without chest pain due to neuropathy. Neuropathy causes impairment or even absence of different sensations, one of them being pain, so the nerves do not transmit pain sensation to the brain to be interpreted. The frequent excess of sugar in the blood destroys nerve endings, causing neuropathy. Of course, that's not to say that diabetics can put their hand on the stove and not scream ouch!

In other cases, diabetics feel chest pain but with the absence of one or more of the other textbook signs and symptoms of a heart attack – for example, pale, sweaty and clammy skin; nausea, vomiting, double incontinence; and fear of impending doom, to name but a few. Jim did not appear to have fear of impending doom; in fact he was very relaxed – exhausted actually, from the convulsing. And he wouldn't have even considered the fact that he may be having a heart attack. Why would he? He didn't have the notorious cardinal sign of chest pain. And silent heart attacks are not common knowledge to the layperson, even to diabetics who know their condition better than most. The pale, sweaty and clammy skin often seen in a patient having a hypoglycaemic episode are the same signs and symptoms generally found in a patient having a heart attack. Hence why a 12 Lead ECG is of paramount importance when attending to any diabetic patient who has high or low blood sugar levels, or who simply complains of feeling unusual or unwell.

I remember an incident I attended to quite a while ago, where the patient was diabetic. He was complaining of feeling very nauseas, so rang treble-nine. While I was undertaking some vital observations on him in the back of the ambulance, we both engaged in some light humour. We were having a great laugh, during which I measured his blood sugar levels. They were off the scale; so high in fact that the glucometer didn't display a decimalised figure, it simply displayed 'HI'. That usually means his blood sugar is above 33mmol/l, although glucometers vary. That's five or six times the norm. So, being thorough, I placed the ECG leads across his chest and one on each limb, while continuing to have a laugh with him. Then, I asked him to refrain from laughing and keep still while the machine analysed his heart rhythm. When the ECG rhythm strip printed, it confirmed he was having a massive heart attack. His only symptom was nausea. No chest pain; no pale, sweaty, clammy skin; no fear of impending doom, just nausea, that's it!

Paramedics carry a clot-busting drug for administration to patients diagnosed by the paramedic as suffering a heart attack. However, a strict set of criteria have to be met by the patient for a paramedic to safely administer the drug. One of the many criteria is chest pain. In order to administer the drug, the patient not only has to meet the strict criteria, but the paramedic has to be absolutely sure a heart attack is occurring.

There's a saying in the medical profession: If it looks like a duck, quacks like a duck and tastes good with orange sauce, then it probably is a duck. Jim looked like a duck (not literally!), but certainly wasn't quacking like one, so I could not be entirely sure that he was having a heart attack. And more to the point, he did not meet the criteria to administer the clot-busting drug, anyway. So, I continued interpreting the ECG rhythm strip, when Gemma interrupted,

'Andy, his blood pressure is one hundred and fifty over eighty-seven. His blood glucose is four. And his temperature is thirty-five point seven.'

'Cheers hun,' I said, placing the ECG strip in my pocket and making a mental note that his blood glucose levels had come up from 2.8mmol/l to 4.0mmol/l. 'Excellent,' I thought, 'maybe it'll continue going in the right direction now.' I then said to Gemma, 'We're gonna have to go through on blues, Gemma, and alert A 'n' E. You go up front an' I'll give you a shout when I'm ready to move off.'

So Gemma stepped out of the back of the ambulance, closed the saloon doors and adopted her position in the driver's seat, and started the engine. I contacted A&E and requested resus to be on standby, and also explained Jim's history behind his presenting condition, my observations, interventions, and an estimated time of arrival. I covered Jim up with several blankets to try and warm him up; he had been so sweaty and clammy that his temperature had dropped. I gave Gemma the nod to mobilise to hospital.

On route, Jim's GCS remained fourteen; the very slight reduction was indicative of confusion as a consequence of his unstable blood sugar levels and convulsing. While Gemma drove us to hospital under emergency driving conditions, I undertook a further blood pressure measurement, which remained similar to his previous one, and a further blood glucose. Alarmingly, his blood sugar was back down to 2.5mmol/l. However, because Jim remained conscious on route, I decided not to administer further IV glucose.

Throughout the journey to hospital, Jim was comfortable but remained pale, sweaty and clammy, regardless of oxygen administration, being wrapped in blankets, or having an adequate blood pressure measurement. When we arrived at the hospital, a doctor and a nurse were ready and waiting to receive my handover and continue assessing and treating Jim. So while we transferred him onto the resuscitation bed, I conveyed my handover to the A&E doctor, which went something like this:

'This is fifty-two year-old Jim. He's type-one insulin diabetic. He has a history of two previous heart attacks and had a coronary artery bypass graft several years ago. Today he skipped breakfast, injected his insulin and then took the dog for a one hour walk, distance unknown.

'At approximately 0930 hours, he went into the bathroom and didn't come out. On our arrival at 0952 hours, I found Jim convulsing. AVPU – U. GCS three. Mouth closed, so nasal airway inserted. Jim was pale, sweaty, clammy and cold to the touch. His temperature is thirty-five point seven. His initial blood glucose was nought point seven.

'Poor IV access choices, but I managed a blue in his right hand, and administered fifty millilitres of ten percent glucose. Blood sugar rose to five point five, but Jim's combative behaviour didn't reflect that, so a further twenty-five millilitres administered. GCS increased to fourteen, but blood glucose reduced again to two point eight. No further glucose administered as he was conscious.

'Respiratory rate sixteen on recovery from seizure. Twelve lead ECG shows some significant changes – query silent MI.

'Blood pressure one hundred and fifty over eighty-seven, and one hundred and fifty-two over ninety, respectively. Blood glucose increased to four before we left scene, but was back down to two point five just prior to arriving here at A 'n' E. GCS has remained fourteen throughout journey, irrespective of his blood sugar level. Are there any questions?'

'No, thank you,' the doctor said. The doctor and nurse immediately began assessing Jim, so Gemma and I went outside to the ambulance to complete the paperwork and refresh the saloon of the vehicle, ready for the next patient.

Later that day in the A&E department, I enquired about Jim's health and wellbeing. The doctor informed me that they had admitted him due to how unstable his blood glucose levels were. He also told me that, having undertaken another ECG in the A&E and comparing their one with mine, it was confirmed that Jim had not suffered a heart attack. The changes on his ECG that I had analysed were probably due to some cardiac ischaemia, which means lack of oxygen to the tissues of the heart, caused by him convulsing. If the changes on the ECG were ischaemia then, once the convulsing had ceased following the administration of glucose and oxygen, the flow of oxygen to Jim's heart must have restored to normal.

Although the back-breaking emergency call given to us as 'a male, diabetic unresponsive' had caught me off guard, and had me twitching a little when I couldn't locate a suitable vein and had anticipated a cardiac arrest would ensue, it had overall been a success. A basic cannula – a very small one – in his hand and a bag of glucose prevented Jim from deteriorating further and falling into cardiac arrest. The equipment and the drugs I used cost pennies, but to Jim and his wife, they were invaluable.

Jim's hypoglycaemia was stabilised during his admission and he was eventually discharged from hospital, but continued to manage his diabetes inadequately due to alcohol. And so, over the following several months, he became well known to ambulance personnel.

Subsequently, six months later, Jim suffered a similar seizure, once again caused by dangerously low blood sugar levels. And although the attending paramedics tried their utmost best to gain IV access in order to administer lifesaving glucose, unfortunately he deteriorated and went into cardiac arrest on scene. The crew rushed him to hospital, performing resuscitation, but Jim failed to respond to treatment after over thirty minutes of cardiac life support, and was sadly pronounced dead in the A&E department a short time later.

Chapter 5
Left for Dead

During the early part of my career as a paramedic, I regularly worked alone, responding to incidents in a Rapid Response Vehicle (RRV). Paramedics *chose* to work alone on an RRV; they were rarely obligated to do so, as solo responding is not every paramedic's cup of tea. Not only can it get quite lonely, but there are also risks attending to incidents with no backup. By backup I mean an extra pair of hands to assist you in both a clinical or confrontational environment. As I mentioned earlier, it's amazing what can be done when there are more than two medical professionals available to attempt to stabilise a dying patient. When working on an RRV, attending to a serious, life-threatening emergency with no immediate backup to assist you, you have to work at speed with just the one pair of hands. Occasionally, you will make use of a member of the public who has offered to assist you, but obviously there's only so much you can ask them to do.

This next incident is a perfect example of what it's like to work alone as a solo responder, with no backup and no member of the public to help out, while attending to a patient who has time-critical and life-threatening injuries. The following incident is a reminder to me of why I joined the ambulance service and what makes me so proud to be a paramedic, when your actions make the difference between life and death.

I was working a twelve hour night shift on an RRV in urban Cheshire one warm summer's night. It was 1:25 a.m. and I was parked up in a lay-by reading a book. As a rule, I could have returned to the ambulance station from midnight onwards, for health and safety purposes. But it had been a very busy night since the start of the shift, for both me and the ambulance crews, so I chose to remain on standby, as I anticipated further treble-nine calls before it quietened down for the rest of the shift.

At 1:30 a.m., the car radio sounded.

'Go ahead,' I said.

'Roger, RED call to an RTC along Terence Lane near Somerton, motorcyclist versus car. The car has left the scene. One patient reported. No vehicles available to assist, all committed. Police attendance requested too, but they've got no one to send at the moment either, over,' the dispatcher said.

'Roger, understood, going mobile, over.'

My first thought was blimey, it's obviously still busy out there; firstly because I was some considerable distance away from the given location, yet I was still the nearest resource for the dispatcher to send. And also because it was highly likely, due to the nature of the call, that the patient was going to need to be conveyed to hospital for further assessment and treatment – so the dispatcher, who I assumed would be thinking the same, would have normally dispatched an ambulance crew. I activated my blue lights, but refrained from using any audible warning devices due to how early in the morning it was, and began mobilising towards the rural location given. The location had a sixty mile per hour speed limit, so a hit-and-run had the potential to be very serious.

On route, I started thinking about the mechanism of potential injuries that can be sustained from a car versus a motorcycle; not that I hadn't dealt with that circumstance before, but that doesn't mean you do not start planning your assessment and potential treatment prior to arriving. Any good paramedic should do that. If you plan for the worst-case scenario, then anything below that is a bonus.

Even with very little traffic to negotiate due to the time of the night, it still took me twenty minutes, with my foot down, to reach the location. A Good Samaritan, a middle-aged woman who had called for the ambulance, approached me as I stepped out of the driver's seat. She had pulled over minutes after the incident occurred, after spotting the motorcycle in her headlights strewn across the tarmac, surrounded by nothing but trees, bushes and foliage. It was pitch black and I could barely see my hand in front of my face. For safety purposes, and to assist the police and ambulance crew in pinpointing my location, I left the blue lights flashing, headlights beaming, and the engine on run-lock to avoid flattening the battery. The environment was eerie and desolate, and if it wasn't for the sound of the engine, you could have heard a pin drop.

I donned my high visibility jacket and protective helmet and liaised with the shaken woman. She pointed out that the motorcyclist was in a ditch and that she could hear him groaning, but was unable to get to him and provide help due to all the undergrowth. By observing where the now written-off motorcycle had come to a halt and where I could hear him groaning, attempting to gain attention, I figured that the motorcyclist had collided with a car and had been knocked off his motorcycle, thrown through the air, and had landed in the undergrowth approximately fifteen to twenty feet away from his machine.

A warm feeling began to stir in my stomach. It was the adrenaline anticipating me having to work at speed, in the dark, with limited space and with no extra hands to assist me.

'What traumatic mess am I going to find in there?' I thought. I grabbed the torch from the RRV, and all of the equipment that I envisaged I might need, including the drugs bag that contained the IV analgesic morphine sulphate and the Entonox – more commonly known as 'gas and air'; that way I wouldn't have to continuously leave the patient unattended and crawl back and forth from the bush where he'd landed.

I shone my torch towards the direction the groaning sound was coming from, while carefully negotiating the uneven ground, ducking underneath and around the protruding branches, occasionally losing my footing and stumbling. After careful negotiation of the terrain, I eventually located the patient and placed my equipment down close by him in order to flatten the branches. I tactfully directed my torch towards the ground, so I could see him yet avoid temporarily blinding him with the bright light. Although the visibility from the torch light wasn't great, I could see that he had removed his helmet himself, and I could see his face. He appeared very grey and sweaty. I immediately suspected that he had sustained a significant injury from the traumatic ordeal.

'Hi mate, my name's Andy, I'm a paramedic. What's y'name?' I asked, taking hold of his wrist to feel for a palpable pulse and rate.

'Car… arrrgh, Carl,' he said, wincing.

'How old are y'Carl?'

'Thirty… thirty-two,' he said with a grimacing expression caused by the excruciating pain he was in from his yet to be identified injuries. I'd felt his pulse throughout and it was racing at 126 bpm. A normal pulse rate for an adult is between 60 and 100 bpm, depending on lifestyle, health or fitness level, etcetera. So I had to assume that Carl's fast pulse rate was due to his body compensating for blood loss.

I must point out that, had I been part of a two-man ambulance crew, I would have immediately took hold of his head and neck to provide manual in-line immobilisation to his c-spine while my crewmate assessed him, or vice versa. C-spine immobilisation is of paramount importance when the mechanism of injury suggests spinal cord damage may have been sustained.

You see, the c-spine cord, or cervical spine cord, is housed and protected by the first seven vertebrae in the spinal column. If the spinal cord suffers damage then the worst-case scenario would be death, but at the very least, most likely leave a victim with life changing disabilities – in other words, paralysed.

The distance Carl had been thrown from his motorcycle meant that he might well have sustained spinal cord injuries. However, because I was a solo responder and he was presenting as grey and sweaty, I had to sacrifice managing his c-spine in order to assess and treat him as fast as possible, as opposed to committing myself solely to in-line immobilisation techniques while I waited for an ambulance crew to arrive.

'OK Carl, I'm just gonna make sure there's an ambulance on route to back me up, and get an ETA on the police as well, mate,' I calmly informed him. I contacted ambulance control via my hand portable radio.

'Ambulance control, go ahead, over.'

'Roger. I need a hot response no divert, to my location, and an ETA on the police too, over.' I couldn't go in to detail as to why I needed hot backup, as Carl would have heard me say that he had the potential for life-threatening injuries. That may have caused him to panic and consequently become irritable, potentially worsening any injuries he had sustained.

'Roger, understood. I still have no vehicles to send at the moment, but I'll send you the next one that clears. The police still have no one to send either. They're very busy too, over.'

'Great,' I thought. 'Roger, understood, over.'

I didn't know how long I was going to be waiting for backup, so I began my questioning, assessment and treatment of Carl, firstly by ascertaining a history of events from him.

'What exactly happened, Carl?'

'I came round the bend and there was a car... on my side of the road… I swerved but he hit me an' I landed 'ere,' he bravely said before pausing due to the sheer pain he was experiencing.

'You're doin' really well, Carl. Just take y'time, mate,' I said reassuringly.

'He stopped an' got out… but then he shouted through the bushes, *sorry mate, I've been drinking*… and then he drove off.'

'What speed was y'both doin'?'

'I wasn't goin' that fast 'cause of the bend. But… he hit me at about fifty, I'd say.'

'OK Carl, I can see you're in a lot of pain. Just bear with me though. I will get rid of your pain, or at least reduce it for you, I promise mate, OK?'

'Yeah… cheers,' he muttered, again with a contorted expression.

I was very impressed with the way Carl handled the pain, as he didn't tend to cry out, just bravely emphasised his sheer agony by verbal pauses and facial expression. The fact that Carl was conversing with me reduced the possibility that he had sustained a significant head injury.

'Right Carl, I just need to do a few tests first, and then I'll need to pop a needle in your hand or arm, so I can give you summot for the pain. I'll be as quick as I can, mate. As far as you're aware, were you knocked out at all?'

'Arrrgh… No.'

'OK, good. Can you tell me where the pain is?'

'My right leg hurts… my thigh and my shin… my right hip… and my back, my lower back I mean.'

'Do you have any pain in y'neck at all?'

'No, just everywhere else,' he said with a brave smile.

'OK. On a scale of zero to ten, how would you score the pain?'

'Ten,' he quickly replied with clear certainty.

I needed to assess Carl quickly, but first needed to begin the process of alleviating his pain, so I initially offered him gas and air, with a view to administering something more potent. The beauty of administering gas and air, also known as 'laughing gas', is that it provides supplemental oxygen to a patient, as well as pain relief; although I had to administer it with caution, as it can be detrimental to a patient if chest injuries are present. So I instructed Carl how to self-administer the laughing gas. Meanwhile, while he was inhaling the gas and air, which contains oxygen, I applied the sats probe to his finger to assess how well oxygenated his blood supply was.

From questioning Carl, and from my first impressions of his grey, sweaty presentation, it was clearly time to start working at speed, as the events leading up to him landing in the bushes meant that he had the potential to deteriorate on me fast! While waiting for the sats monitor to display a measurement, I removed my tuffcut scissors from my trouser leg pocket, and with haste cut the right sleeve of his leather motorcycle jacket, and his shirt, so I could undertake a blood pressure measurement.

The reason measuring his blood pressure was a priority over administering any intravenous pain relief – for instance, morphine sulphate – was because a patient's systolic blood pressure has to be above 90mmHg to meet the criteria for a paramedic to safely administer morphine; morphine can reduce blood pressure if a significant amount of internal or external haemorrhaging is present. If his blood pressure was already low and I administered morphine, it could reduce considerably, to below a level that is required to sustain life, and consequently kill him.

My only option would be to administer intravenous fluid in order to keep his blood pressure high enough to sustain a systolic of 90mmHg or above, in the event that any morphine I administered did significantly reduce it. However, as mentioned in the first chapter, the body has a natural defence mechanism to clot haemorrhaging. Administering fluid can encourage clots to dilute and break down, therefore causing haemorrhaging to recommence, so I had to be very careful and monitor him closely throughout… with just a torch for light.

The sats monitor displayed a measurement of ninety-seven percent while on gas and air. That was good enough for me! So I applied the blood pressure cuff to his right arm, took out my stethoscope – an acoustic medical device for listening to sounds in the human body – and inflated the cuff. But I was unable to clearly see the dial on the monitor, because of the poor light. I tried to move the torch around to gain a clearer view, but that proved useless, so instead resorted to placing my pen-torch – which is primarily used to assess the eyes' pupillary response to light – into my mouth and depressed the button with my teeth, so I could clearly see the needle on the dial. After several seconds of deflating the cuff and listening for the appropriate sounds, I obtained a blood pressure measurement of 100/60mmHg.

That blood pressure measurement was a crucial observation. He was thirty-two years old, and even though a systolic blood pressure of 100mmHg can be normal for a thirty-two year-old, it is rare, especially when in severe pain. I had to presume that his fast pulse rate and low blood pressure were indicative of significant bleeding somewhere. There was no evidence of external bleeding from what I could see with the torch, so I suspected internal bleeding only.

With a blood pressure measurement obtained, I deflated the remainder of the air left in the cuff, but left it wrapped around his arm with a view to further measurements while waiting for backup. Carl continued to self-administer the gas and air, but he was still evidently experiencing a lot of pain, judging by the audible moans and groans he was making. I began considering my next task of cannulating. I used the torch to locate the cannulation equipment from the paramedic bag, and then once again inflated the blood pressure cuff still wrapped around his right arm, to improvise a tourniquet. The veins of his right hand swelled with venous blood. That was a positive sign that he wasn't rapidly shutting down from blood loss, which subsequently causes veins to 'collapse', making cannulation very difficult. It was going to be difficult enough in the pitch black with just a pen-torch in my mouth, without having to struggle to find a vein too!

I removed the long, wide needle from its packaging and placed my pen-torch into my mouth to direct some light on Carl's right hand, so I didn't miss the vein. Taking hold of his arm, I pierced the skin and entered the vein with the needle. The flashback quickly appeared in the chamber. I advanced further and waited for a secondary flashback along the length of the clear plastic tube. That too appeared. Then, I removed the 'tourniquet' and applied digital pressure to the vein, withdrew the needle, and discarded the needle into the sharps container. I screwed the Luer-Lock to the end and quickly flushed the cannula with a pre-filled syringe of sodium chloride, and secured the patent IV access point with an adhesive dressing.

I now needed to quickly assess for injuries, prior to preparing and administering morphine, so I used my tuffcut scissors to cut his right and left boots off, assessed for a palpable pulse in his foot, and marked it with an 'X'. That was done to signify to the hospital doctors that a pulse *distal* – meaning the farthest point of his leg from the fracture site – was confirmed. The absence of a palpable distal pedal pulse can be indicative of a reduced blood supply to the limb, which can therefore be limb threatening.

Carl was still groaning, in between periods of self-administering the gas and air. Although I was well aware that he was in a lot of pain, I needed to assess what injuries he had, as they would determine how I managed his pain and what risk factors I had to take into account. I cut his jeans from the bottom, right up to the top and through his belt, on both the left and the right side. Then, I slowly directed the light of the torch towards his lower limbs, scanning both sides from the bottom of his shins, right up to the top of his thigh. There was an obvious deformity in his right shinbones (tibia and fibula) and in his right femur (thighbone). You didn't need to be Superman with X-ray vision to figure that his femur, tibia and fibula were fractured; it was blatantly noticeable. Fortunately, they were all closed fractures, but nonetheless very serious, particularly the femur.

Femur fractures, whether open or closed, are time-critical, as death can occur if major arteries are ruptured. If the site of the ruptured artery is not located and 'clamped', as it were, in a timely manner, the patient may bleed to death. I was also concerned that he had a fractured pelvis too – which often, not always, goes hand-in-hand with a fractured femur – because he had stated that his lower back was hurting. That complaint can be indicative of a fractured pelvis, but to assess it in any way could be detrimental and potentially worsen the prognosis. I therefore focused on the injuries that I had identified. Pain relief and keeping him stable were my priorities for this severely injured motorcyclist, in the absence of an ambulance crew to assist me in splinting and immobilising his fractured limbs, and furthermore, in what would ideally have been the application of full c-spine immobilisation equipment.

I encouraged Carl to continue self-administering the gas and air, and reassured him that a more potent and effective analgesia was imminent. At the same time, I hastily, yet carefully, began preparing the morphine and a drug called metoclopramide – an anti-nausea/sickness drug – once again with the pen-torch lit between my teeth.

I made the decision to administer an anti-sickness drug to Carl as morphine can often cause nausea or vomiting, and I didn't want him vomiting while he was not only in a lot of pain, but also because of the injuries he had sustained. He may also have sustained injuries that I was unable to confirm while situated in undergrowth, and in the pitch black. Also, because the mechanism of his injuries – by that I mean colliding with a car and being thrown through the air, landing some distance away from his motorcycle – had the potential to cause spinal cord injuries, the last thing I wanted was him rolling around if he began vomiting. Clearly, keeping still is the preferred treatment for a patient whose mechanism of injury has the potential for a spinal cord injury.

After a few minutes of preparation, the drugs were drawn up into syringes and ready for me to administer.

'Right Carl, how would you score your pain now, while using the gas 'n' air?' I asked.

'Bad… about a nine,' he replied, once again with a contorted expression.

'OK, I'm gonna give you an anti-sickness drug first, alright? Then I'll give y'some morphine, OK?'

'Arrrgh… Yeah,' he replied, grimacing. So I slowly, over a period of two minutes, pushed the anti-sickness drug through the cannula and into his veins, before flushing the drug through with a small amount of sodium chloride. I encouraged Carl to keep self-administering the gas and air while I slowly administered an initial five milligram dose of morphine, as that would provide additional pain relief, followed by a further small amount of sodium chloride to push the drug through. While waiting to see if the first dose of morphine had any effect on his pain score, and using the torch clamped between my legs at an angle for light, I quickly prepared a five hundred millilitre bag of sodium chloride. I then attached it to the cannula, hung the bag from a branch and opened up the clamp slightly, so the fluid dripped at a slow rate.

It was now imperative that I undertook a second blood pressure measurement to see if the morphine, combined with obvious internal bleeding, had caused his blood pressure to drop. So placed the pen-torch in my mouth again and measured his blood pressure. It was by now reading 90/50mmHg; a slight reduction was noted.

'What would you say your pain score is now, Carl?'

'Seven,' he said, still grimacing. I palpated for a pulse in his wrist it was still present. As there was still no sign of the ambulance crew I'd requested some thirty minutes ago, nor had the police arrived either, I administered a further two point five milligram of morphine, with extreme caution.

While waiting for the ambulance, I frequently monitored Carl's conscious level, pulse rate and pain score – which gradually reduced to a five out of ten – and undertook an initial blood glucose level. To my alarm, when I measured Carl's blood pressure for the third time, it had diminished considerably. The morphine I had given him, along with his internal bleeding, had reduced it significantly; it was now measuring just 75/45mmHg.

I felt for a pulse again, in his wrist. It was impalpable. I had no choice but to open up the clamp of the drip fully, allowing the contents to run rapidly. I thought about obtaining a secondary IV access point in his left hand or arm. This is encouraged by doctors in certain circumstances, particularly in major trauma or if you have no choice but to remain on scene with a patient – just the situation I was in here. I thought against it. As long as I could keep his blood pressure adequate, I was happy with just the one IV access point I'd already secured.

I had been on scene, out in the sticks, for nearly an hour, when suddenly I saw blue flashing lights through the gaps in the bushes It was an ambulance crew. And to no surprise, a couple of minutes after the ambulance had arrived, the traffic police arrived too.

'Typical,' I thought, 'just like buses!'

One member of the ambulance crew fought their way through the foliage to assist and liaise with me, while his crewmate fetched the spinal immobilisation equipment, including the longboard, rather like a rigid stretcher on to which a patient suspected of having spinal cord injuries can be immobilised and secured. He then battled his way through the bushes too. Between the three of us, we applied a box splint to Carl's fractured leg, fully immobilised him on to the longboard, and then began fighting through the bushes until we negotiated our way out of the logistically challenging location. We eventually got back on to the tarmac of the road, where the stretcher had been positioned for Carl's imminent exit from the undergrowth.

We placed the longboard onto the stretcher. I hastily placed my equipment back into the rear of the RRV and then stepped into the saloon of the ambulance, where the crew was just securing the stretcher in place. Now that artificial light was present, I could clearly see how pale and sweaty Carl appeared. He was still very clammy to the touch, too, and evidently still in pain, even after seven point five milligram of morphine and almost continual gas and air. The crew began cutting the remainder of Carl's clothes off, in order to expose and examine for other less obvious injuries. They then undertook a further blood pressure measurement, attached the ECG leads to him, and assessed his pupillary response.

Meanwhile, I liaised with the police officer, informing him of what Carl had told me of the driver's words to him through the bushes, admitting to drinking before he'd driven off, leaving Carl injured, alone and left for dead in the ditch. I also enlightened him as to the life-threatening injuries Carl had sustained, and what hospital he would be taken to.

I once again stepped back into the saloon of the ambulance, where the crew was undertaking further observations on Carl.

'What's his blood pressure now, mate?' I asked inquisitively.

'Eighty-five over sixty, mate.'

'Excellent, it's come up a bit with the fluid then.' I took hold of Carl's wrist again, while looking at the ECG monitor displaying a heart rate and rhythm. A pulse was palpable and the ECG rate was 120 bpm. Carl was still compensating very well and the fluid had achieved what I had intended, although it had by now depleted, so I attached a further bag to the fluid giving set and opened it very slightly.

I then contacted the A&E department direct, to inform them of Carl's age, history of events, the mechanism that caused his injuries, what injuries I had diagnosed, vital signs, other potential injuries, treatment provided, and the estimated time of his arrival. That would ensure a trauma team could be alerted and awaiting Carl's arrival, and have a reasonably clear understanding of what they would be shortly receiving. I then informed ambulance control that I was going to travel in the back of the ambulance with Carl to A&E, and that my colleague would drive the RRV through to A&E for me. It made sense, as I had ascertained the history of events from Carl and had spent the best part of an hour with him, and had provided the treatment, so was able to give an educated and detailed handover to the awaiting doctors on arrival at A&E.

Carl was conveyed to hospital under emergency driving conditions. While on route he remained very calm and quiet, and although his pain score had reduced, his facial expressions suggested he was still uncomfortable. I continued to monitor his blood pressure, pulse rate and his GCS, which remained at fifteen throughout.

When we arrived inside the resus room, a trauma team was gloved, gowned and ready to accept Carl and continue with his assessment and treatment. So as several members of the team transferred him from the ambulance stretcher onto the awaiting resus bed, I gave them the information they required; it went something like this:

'This is Carl, he's thirty-two years old. At approximately 0125 hours he was hit by a car at approximately fifty mile per hour and landed approximately fifteen to twenty feet away from his machine, on reasonably soft terrain in some bushes. On arrival, Carl was grey, sweaty and clammy. His sats were ninety-seven percent on gas 'n' air.

'He is complaining of lower back pain, right hip pain, right femur pain and right shin pain. No complaints of neck pain, although we've immobilised him due to the mechanism of his injuries.

'Carl removed his helmet himself prior to my arrival. C-spine not immediately immobilised because I was on my own. I'm confident he's got a right fractured femur and right fractured tibia and fibula as there is obvious deformity. Pedal pulse palpable and marked with an 'X'. Right leg box splinted. He has a query pelvic injury, too.

'On examination, AVPU – A. GCS fifteen throughout. Exact respiratory rate not measured, but no breathing concerns noted. Blood glucose normal. He initially had a palpable radial pulse. Pulse rate initially one hundred and twenty-six, but now approximately one hundred and twenty. Pain score initially ten out of ten pre-analgesia, now five post seven point five milligram of morphine in addition to gas 'n' air. No further morphine administered.

'Blood pressure initially one hundred over sixty. Now fluctuating between eighty-five and ninety, post morphine. A five hundred mil fluid challenge initially administered but depleted, so a second bag attached, but I have only kept the clamp slightly open to maintain a palpable radial pulse. On crew arrival, patient fully immobilised and extracted from foliage. Are there any questions?'

'No, thank you,' the lead doctor replied. The trauma team then began assessing Carl, measuring his blood pressure again, before giving him further pain relief or fluid.

By the time I had completed my paperwork, the night had become a little calmer, and a little lighter, too! I only had a few hours of my shift left to go, so I got the RRV keys back off my colleague and headed back to the station for a well-earned brew.

While off duty a few days later, I received a telephone call from the police, requesting a statement. So, although not normal practice, I invited a police officer around to my home – statements can and often do take two to three hours to complete, and are therefore not always practical to undertake while on duty. The main reason the police wanted a statement from me was that I was a key witness for Carl, simply because of what he had told me at the scene about the driver. While giving my statement, the police officer informed me that he had been in contact with the ward doctors that were looking after Carl, and had been told by them that Carl was extremely lucky to be alive. Had it not been for the passing motorist spotting the wreckage of Carl's motorcycle a short time after the collision and stopping to investigate, he would have gone unfound for some time. He would have bled to death from his injuries.

A couple of months later, I received a letter in the post requesting me to advise of any dates that I would not be available to attend court, if required as a witness. This would have been necessary in the event that the driver, who had been arrested in the early hours of that morning, did not plead guilty at his upcoming court appearance. Fortunately, he did plead guilty and was given a custodial sentence for driving over the legal alcohol limit, dangerous driving, and leaving the scene of a collision.

Fortunately, Carl had not sustained a spinal cord injury, but did spend several months in hospital with fractures to his right femur (thighbone), tibia and fibula (shin bones), right hip, pelvis and left shoulder. Although not permanently disabled, Carl would not walk normally, without pain, discomfort or limitations, for a considerable period of time.

The Dark Side

Chapter 6
A Fateful Decision

Being a paramedic is not *rocket science*. Ninety percent of the job involves being able to listen and have excellent communication and inter-personal skills. The other ten percent is clinical knowledge. It's as easy as ABC – Airway, Breathing and Circulation. You do not move on to Breathing until you have secured a patent Airway; which may involve the use of airway adjuncts. And you do not move on to Circulation until you have confirmed the patient is adequately Breathing, or until you are ventilating them either manually or by mechanical means, such as an automatic ventilator.

The most difficult part of the job is maintaining the physiological knowledge and correlating that to the patient's presenting signs and symptoms, history of events, and vital signs undertaken while in your care. Then applying that knowledge, combined with risk assessments and clinical thought processes, to arrive at an appropriate treatment plan and care pathway. Furthermore, paramedics are not always obliged to diagnose a condition with accuracy – although we often do. We are merely expected to treat what we see, and if required, convey the patient to definitive care. Here a doctor or doctors will endeavour to diagnose the patient's condition with further comparative observations and assessments not available in the pre-hospital setting; for example, blood tests, x-rays, Computerised Tomography (CT) scans, Magnetic Resonance Imaging (MRI), etcetera.

Case in point: the following incident I attended to is a perfect example of treating what you see, as opposed to accurately diagnosing a condition. It was 2 a.m. and I was half way through a night shift on a cold winter's morning. My crewmate, John, an experienced ambulance technician, was resting his eyes in another room of the ambulance station, and I was sat up with another paramedic watching TV for insomniacs, or night shift workers!

The non-emergency telephone rang, and with me being the closest to the telephone and the next in line to go out, I answered it.

John and I were dispatched to an eighteen year-old male with D and V (diarrhoea and vomiting); that was the only information I received from the ambulance dispatcher. The call was triaged by the ambulance control room call-taker as an urgent response, which means the caller rang treble-nine but, following questioning, was found to be non-life-threatening, so blue lights and audible warning devices were therefore not required – not that I would use them at 2 a.m. in the morning, unless absolutely necessary, of course.

So off we went in the direction of the given address, which was in quite a rural part of Cheshire, about twelve miles away from the ambulance station I was working from. We were only moving at a snail's pace because it wasn't a blue light call, the road conditions were quite slippery... and John was driving. John was a funny character, horizontal in nature and a very likable bloke. I remember a very funny incident involving him; in fact I remember a lot of funny incidents involving him, but I'll just tell you this one.

John was on a day shift one very hot summer's day, driving back from the A&E department to the ambulance station. His crewmate was reading the paper in the attendant's seat. They were comfortably ambling along when they stumbled upon a traffic jam on a long, straight road. It was so congested that John turned the engine off; they were going nowhere.

An hour went by and John's crewmate was all of a sudden startled at the sound of periodic car horns. He then realised he'd nodded off while reading the paper, due to the scorching temperature and lack of any breeze entering the cab. Still stationary, he looked ahead and noticed there was no longer congested traffic. He turned to ask John, sat in the driver's seat, why they were still stationary even though the traffic was no longer jammed... only to find John fast asleep too. For about ten minutes, motorists had been driving around them, beeping their horns at John's thoughtless and inconsiderate parking in the left-hand lane of a busy road. Fantastic! You couldn't write it for a sitcom, could you!

Anyway, when we eventually arrived at the front door of the patient's address with equipment to hand and entered the property, a lady beckoned us to go upstairs. As we reached the top of the staircase, we were greeted by the lady I rightly assumed was the patient's mother. At the same time, the patient, a teenager, came out of the bathroom wearing a bathrobe. He appeared pale, sweaty and dazed, almost like he was sleepwalking. The foul stench from the bathroom suddenly attacked my nasal passages. It was nauseating to say the least, even with my bowels of iron constitution. I remember thinking, if you could bottle that odour and sell it to the army, you'd make a fortune. However, he didn't even acknowledge that we were stood at the top of the stairs; he just walked into his bedroom, climbed back into bed, rolled over towards the wall and threw the covers over himself. I looked at his mum, who had contacted the ambulance service; she gazed back at me, concerned,

'I'm sorry for wasting your time, I know you're busy. I was going to leave him to sleep and just get the doctor out when they're open in the morning, but that's hours away and I was worried. I'm so sorry,' she said.

'No, don't apologise. Tell me what your concern is, my love.'

'Well, he's been unwell for a couple of days with cold like symptoms, and all day yesterday, and throughout the night, he's had vomiting and diarrhoea. He's acting really strange, confused like, ya know, and not responding properly when I try talkin' to him,' she explained.

'OK, what's his name, love?'

'Matthew, Matt,' she informed me.

I sat on the edge of the bed and shook Matt's shoulder while calling his name; he just shrugged off my attempts at trying to get him to roll over and face me so I could talk to him. So I left him as he was while I took hold of his wrist to feel for a pulse, which was strong and evidently present.

'It's fast… must be a hundred and forty at least,' I said, looking at John. 'Matt! Matt! Can you turn around and face me please, mate?' No response. 'Matt! Matt!' He turned and faced me. He looked awful. His eyes appeared drawn and tired, and his skin was pasty. 'How do you feel? And don't say with your hands,' I asked, hoping to gain a humorous grin from him. No smile, no grin.

'Rough,' he muttered. I felt his forehead.

'He feels very warm and clammy,' I said, directing my eyes towards his mum. I opened the paramedic bag and reached for the oxygen saturations monitor and thermometer, to measure how well his blood was oxygenated, and his temperature. His sats were ninety-six percent. 'That's pretty good,' I thought, 'but not quite right for a young, fit lad.' His temperature measured 38.7°C. That's a high fever. By now my concerns were beginning to heighten because a heart rate of 140 bpm, in addition to a fever and D and V, was not good, a sure sign of infection.

'OK Matt, I just need to take your blood pressure, check your blood sugar levels and administer a little oxygen. You stay lying down, OK mate?'

I asked John to set up the oxygen and then measure Matt's blood glucose. Meanwhile, I rolled up the sleeve of his bathrobe and wrapped the cuff of the blood pressure monitor around the upper aspect of his right arm, inflated it and placed my stethoscope midway up his arm, where the brachial pulse is. I listened carefully for the appropriate audible sounds heard when measuring blood pressure.

'Umm… it's very low. I know he's young and slim but it's lower than it should be,' I said, looking at his mum. Matt's systolic blood pressure measured 100mmHg.

What Matt's body was in fact doing was compensating. Because his blood pressure was low, his heart was beating faster to pump and circulate blood around the body in order to adequately oxygenate the vital organs, a sure physiological sign of shock – exactly what type of shock I wasn't sure of at this point. However, I knew something was seriously wrong and I was becoming increasingly concerned.

'What's his blood sugar, mate?' I asked John, while thinking about my observations so far.

'Normal,' John replied.

'His GCS is fluctuating between thirteen and fourteen,' I began pondering to myself, 'he's got a high temp; he's sweaty; he's acting intermittently dazed; he's got a rapid heart rate; his blood pressure is low, and he's had vomiting and diarrhoea.' I began to get a bit of a gut feeling. 'OK Matt, would you mind opening your bathrobe and let me assess the colour of your body… is that OK, mate?' He didn't answer; he just opened up the robe and exposed the front of his body, leaving the boxer shorts he was wearing in place. I then, very carefully and meticulously, scanned the appearance of his skin. His chest, stomach and legs looked pale and mottled, particularly his legs.

Mottled skin can be a normal presentation when a person has a fever, chest infection, common cold or other non-life-threatening condition, but with Matt's presenting signs and symptoms I wasn't going to take any risks whatsoever. I turned to his mum,

'I know it might sound like a silly question but I have to ask; has he had any surgery lately or been out of the country? Or around anyone who has been out of the country, or anybody that's still ill or that has been ill?' I asked, like it was the Spanish inquisition.

'Er... one of his friends has just come back from France; they had the flu while they were there. But he's not had any operations or anything, no,' she replied.

'Matt, is your neck stiff at all, or does the bedroom light hurt your eyes?' I inquisitively asked.

'No... I've got 'ed-ache though,' he mumbled, as if he didn't have the energy to even speak. I stood up from the edge of the bed and faced Matt's mum,

'I'll be upfront and honest with you, Matt's not very well at all. I think he might have meningococcal septicaemia and we need to get him to hospital fast. If I'm wrong then great, but until proven otherwise I'll treat him for what I can see. He's not got the notorious rash as such, but his skin does appear to be mottled. So, we'll get him on the ambulance, pop a needle into his arm and give him some IV fluid and benzyl penicillin. He's not allergic to penicillin, is he?'

'No... he's not, no,' she answered with an understandably concerned expression.

Now, before I continue, let me explain a little about meningococcal septicaemia, a condition that kills approximately 1500 people in the UK every year. Meningococcal septicaemia is a form of blood poisoning caused by a specific bacterium, and patients often develop a rash, but the rash is usually at a late stage. The bacteria cause damage to the blood vessels, allowing blood to leak out under the skin. This causes a rash of red or purple bruises, or sometimes blood blisters, which can appear anywhere on the body. If a glass tumbler is pressed firmly against the rash it will not fade and you will still be able to see the rash through the glass.

The mottled skin I observed on Matt's chest, stomach and legs during my assessment can, and often does, rapidly become a purpuric rash, sometimes within minutes; death is imminent without effective antibiotic treatment, and the earlier the antibiotics are administered, the better the chances are of the patient surviving. Let me repeat that sentence again: the earlier the antibiotics are administered, the better the chances are of the patient surviving.

Now, you may remember earlier I mentioned that Mr X, my paramedic instructor, and I would sometimes end up in a heated debate over the treatment I had given to my fictitious patient, and that I would stand my ground; especially when what I had done wasn't necessarily wrong or detrimental to the patient. I'd simply deviated a little from the JRCALC guidelines – a paramedic's bible – for the benefit of my patient. Well, this was a typical example of deviating from the guidelines – not necessarily one that Mr X and I had debated about during my paramedic course, but it is an example of why I would occasionally deviate from my 'bible'.

You see, the indications for the administration of benzyl penicillin, in the edition of the JRCALC guidelines I was working to during this particular incident, stated: *if the rash is not present, then treat the shock and keep looking for the rash.* In other words, DO NOT administer benzyl penicillin until you can see the rash. I wasn't prepared to take that risk. They are, after all, only guidelines and not protocols, and although I hadn't diagnosed Matt as having meningococcal septicaemia, there had already been a delay in his treatment. If his presenting signs and symptoms were eventually diagnosed as meningococcal septicaemia, I'd be devastated if I hadn't administered antibiotics early.

I couldn't help but feel a little annoyed at the fact that we could have been at Matt's bedside thirty or forty minutes earlier, had the call been triaged appropriately as an emergency, and consequently John had driven a little faster. We would've been well on our way to A&E by now. The information obtained by the ambulance call-taker from Matt's mum had not been adequate enough to triage the call as an emergency blue light response. The delay, from the time Matt's mum made the treble-nine call to arriving at hospital, could now make the difference between life and death. I don't believe it was the call-taker's fault; in my opinion, I think it was a flaw in the triage process which at the time of writing this book has since become obsolete – although, even today, triage errors do occur, but fortunately are rare.

I asked John to go and get the carry chair as I didn't want Matt walking down the stairs to the ambulance, he was far too unwell. Based on my questioning, assessment and findings so far, his condition was time-critical, whether he had meningococcal septicaemia or not; he was in shock and would soon die if not treated with the utmost urgency.

When John arrived back in the bedroom with the carry chair, Matt moved from his bed and sat himself down, with a little assistance from us. We quickly but carefully carried him down the stairs and wheeled him across the gravelled driveway and into the back of the ambulance, and assisted him in to a semi-recumbent position on the stretcher. I placed a blanket over him, taking into consideration that he had a high temperature and therefore I didn't want to unnecessarily overheat him further. I directed Matt's mum to a seat, so she could travel with us to the hospital as opposed to following in her own car. I reassured her that the appropriate treatment would begin imminently, as she was obviously beside herself with worry.

'Right John, contact ambulance control and tell 'em to alert A 'n' E resus. We've got an eighteen year-old male, GCS thirteen stroke fourteen, rapid heart rate, high temperature, low blood pressure and mottled skin. Tell 'em meningococcal septicaemia cannot be ruled out,' I said with an obvious and clear sense of urgency. 'Oh and tell 'em I'm going to administer IV benzyl penicillin. Then get us in on blue lights as steady as y'can, please mate.'

John conveyed the pre-alert message to ambulance control and then began mobilising to A&E. I quickly attached the ECG leads to Matt, to observe his exact heart rate and rhythm, and then undertook another blood pressure reading, this time using the automatic method in order to leave my hands free and progress with my treatment by cannulating him.

Matt's ECG rhythm was normal for a young, fit lad, but his heart rate was now 146 bpm and he wasn't even exerting himself; that is not a good sign at all, whatsoever. The second blood pressure reading was also showing a figure even lower than what I had measured in the bedroom. While that can be normal, particularly in a moving ambulance, it can also be due to deterioration; Matt was potentially a short time away from irreversible shock and ultimately death.

I started preparing the equipment to cannulate Matt and then asked John to pull the ambulance over, so I could safely cannulate him without the risk of missing his vein or stabbing him, or me, with a sharp needle. In the event, John drove over a hump, pothole or round a bend as I was piercing the skin. I quickly cannulated and secured the plastic tube in place, then hurriedly prepared an adult dosage of the drug, benzyl penicillin, as I didn't want John stationary for too long. I gave John the nod that the drug was prepared and I was no longer playing with sharp needles. He moved off again and continued the journey to the hospital under blue light conditions, carefully negotiating the slippery roads.

Matt was by now becoming increasingly agitated and lethargic, positioned semi-recumbent on the stretcher. I asked him again if I could assess his skin colour. With a dazed expression, he consented with a nod of his head. He didn't even have the energy to talk. He was deteriorating. So I scanned his torso and lower limbs again, and to my alarm the mottling had worsened; it appeared to be more noticeable than it had in the house just a short time ago.

With the powdered drug now dissolved in water and contained in a syringe, I pushed it through the cannula and into Matt's veins, before setting up a bag of sodium chloride fluid and attaching that to the cannula, allowing the contents to run freely. While travelling along the deserted roads at an ungodly hour, I continued to closely monitor Matt's torso and limbs for further deterioration, in addition to undertaking further heart rate and blood pressure measurements. His mum was becoming increasingly concerned, so I repeatedly reassured her that we would soon be at hospital and the doctors would see Matt immediately, without delay.

When we arrived at the A&E resus department and had wheeled Matt into the hospital, John escorted Matt's mum to the relatives' room. A doctor and two nurses had donned protective gloves, gowns and face masks as a result of me asking John to mention to ambulance control that meningococcal septicaemia could not be ruled out; the message had been successfully conveyed, thus protecting the doctors and nurses from cross infection. It was too late for us, we'd already been exposed.

We quickly transferred Matt from our stretcher to the resus bed; cue my ungrammatical handover to the doctor, which went something like this:

'This is Matt, eighteen years old. No significant past medical history; no known allergies. He's had common cold like symptoms for two days, and for the last eighteen hours or so has had D and V. Matt has been around a friend who had flu like symptoms in France recently.

'On arrival, AVPU – V. Matt appeared dazed, sweaty, clammy and complaining of headache. No complaints of stiff neck or dislike of bright lights, though. On examination, his GCS was intermittently thirteen stroke fourteen throughout. Respiratory rate fifteen.

'His pulse is running at approximately one hundred and fifty beats per minute, but his ECG rhythm and glucose levels are normal. His systolic blood pressure was initially one hundred but decreased, so a five hundred millilitre fluid challenge administered. Temperature was thirty-eight point seven.

'He has gradually worsening mottled skin to chest, stomach and legs. O-two administered. IV access gained and one point two grams of benzyl penicillin administered as a precaution. Current blood pressure is one hundred and ten systolic. Are there any questions?'

The doctors had no questions for me. They immediately began taking repeat comparative measurements of the tests I had done, to assess for improved or worsening signs and symptoms. They then took blood samples from Matt to test for a number of bacterium, in order to confirm meningococcal septicaemia or another cause of his time-critical presentation. Matt was now in the expert hands of the doctors.

Due to Matt's potential diagnosis, we had to return to the station to change ambulances so the one we had used to convey him to hospital could be deep cleaned by a private infection control valeting company. So we returned to the ambulance station for a much needed brew, and to check out a spare vehicle too.

A short time later, we were dispatched to another treble-nine, and upon arriving at the A&E with a little, frail old lady who had fallen and sustained a fractured wrist, I was approached by the doctor I had earlier handed Matt over to. He informed me that, about twenty minutes after I had left the hospital, Matt's body was absolutely covered in a purpuric, non-blanching rash, and so he was swiftly transferred to the Intensive Care Unit (ICU) of the hospital. Meningococcal septicaemia was the cause.

Later that morning, while at home in bed, I received an urgent telephone call from the ambulance station manager, asking me to visit the hospital. A doctor had prescribed all those who had come in to contact with Matt, a preventative dose of antibiotics, because we were all at risk of infection from any potential droplets sprayed from Matt's bodily fluids, such as saliva from coughing, or mucous from a sneeze.

Several weeks later, upon me enquiring, I found out that Matt had survived, although he had sustained some temporary after effects caused by the bacterial infection. However, if Matt's mum had not made that fateful decision to call for an ambulance when she did, and instead left him alone to sleep, undisturbed, and waited until the doctors' surgery opened some five or so hours later as she'd initially planned, the outcome would have been very different. Matt, without a doubt, would have died.

Chapter 7
An Undignified Death

Suicide: cowardly or courageous?

It's subjective, isn't it? On one hand, it takes nerves of steel to end your own life with the knowledge that you will never see your loved ones ever again, nor will they ever see you again, either... unless you believe in an afterlife, that is. On the other hand, it signifies a weakness to continue fighting, to battle through life regardless of what it throws at you, against any odds. I personally don't think I'd have the guts or selfishness to kill myself. Although, until faced with an extremely difficult predicament, who can ever be sure of what they would be capable of under extreme circumstances?

During my career in the ambulance service, I've attended to hundreds of patients who have attempted suicide, and most of the time it was a *cry for help* – that's not my unsympathetic opinion, most actually admit it if you ask them outright. And in the majority of cases they knew they'd neither taken enough pills nor slashed their wrists deep enough, or in the right direction, to kill themselves. And why would you call an ambulance if you genuinely intended to kill yourself? You wouldn't, would you!

The genuine suicides I've attended to hadn't changed their minds after the deed was initiated. They were found dead by a family member; a spouse, a sibling, a parent, or occasionally a member of the public. On one occasion, an hotelier found a resident lying face down on the bed in his hotel room, with a detailed and well written suicide letter next to him, explaining his exact reasons for taking his own life. He had taken an overdose of prescription codeine. Unfortunately, he turned out to be the partner of a colleague of mine. I never did tell her that it was me who had attended to him and confirmed him dead.

Of the handful of genuinely successful suicides I've dealt with as a paramedic, the most unpleasant one of them all was on a Christmas Eve morning several years ago. It was 6 a.m. and the night had been extremely busy for all of the ambulance crews on the out-station I was working from. Like other crews, my mate, Mike, and I had dealt with unconscious or injured party revellers pretty much since 8 p.m. the previous evening, as you might expect the majority of the UK Ambulance Service to do, two joyful, party-going nights before Christmas morning. I was exhausted and had just two hours left until I could go home and inspect the inside of my eyelids.

We were sat in the station mess room surrounded by festive decorations, clock watching, hoping not to be called out again for the remainder of the shift, as we'd had more than enough verbal abuse and drunken frivolities for one night... and we'd be back for more of it in just fourteen hours time. Unfortunately, at 6:20 a.m., my hand portable radio sounded.

'Go ahead, over.'

'Roger, respond cold to Graysfield Road near Memorial Bridge; a pedestrian has reported a man hanging. Police and Fire on route also, over.'

'Did I hear right then, a man hanging from the bridge?' I asked Mike.

'I think so,' he replied.

'Roger, understood, over,' I replied.

My first thought was that this is not going to be as given. Hanging my arse! On Christmas Eve morning, no chance! This is going to be a drunken hoax – which was common. So Mike and I reluctantly moved from our warm, cosy armchairs and went outside into the cold, dark environment once again.

We trundled along in the ambulance to the given location, which was only five minutes' drive away from the ambulance station. As we rolled up to the scene, we suddenly came across an eerie figure hanging from the bridge, about twenty feet or so up in the air, above double spiked security railings. The pedestrian's grim discovery was not the Christmas Eve hoax I had anticipated. A copper was already on scene and awaiting our presence, not that he would have been expecting us to do anything remotely lifesaving, just waiting to liaise with us.

My eyes had slightly adapted to the dark during the short journey, and I could see the grey figure swinging as the breeze pushed it side to side. For about twenty seconds or so, Mike and I just sat there gawping at it. It was a surreal moment, like something from a movie, as neither of us had attended a hanging before – not one that was still swinging anyway; they've usually been cut down by the person who discovered it by the time an ambulance crew arrives, and they're normally indoors, too. This hanging was in full public view, and also too high to consider immediate recovery, as he had chosen, whether deliberately or not, the Long Drop method of hanging.

Now, before I continue with the story, allow me to explain to you the mechanism behind suicide by the Long Drop method of hanging. The Long Drop method breaks the neck by the body falling and then being brought up with a sharp jerk by the rope. At the end of the drop, the body is still accelerating under the force of gravity but the head is constrained by the noose.

The only difference with this bloke was he chose to hang himself with a freight strap, with a hook connector attached, as opposed to a rope. He had positioned the hook connector slightly to the left of the angle of his jaw – intentional or not, we'll never know, but that would usually cause the head to rotate backwards. This, combined with the downward momentum of the body, breaks the neck and ruptures the spinal cord, causing instant, deep unconsciousness and rapid death. It is only in the last six inches or so of the drop that the physical damage to the neck occurs, as the rope constricts the neck and the force is applied to the vertebrae.

So, after twenty seconds or so of gawping at the unnerving, suspended figure, we stepped out of the ambulance and approached the copper to liaise with him. While stood talking, we all kept repeatedly looking up at the body. I don't know why, I can only assume it was morbid curiosity emerging, and also because there was nothing we could do other than hang around (pardon the pun) and wait for the Fire Brigade to arrive in an appliance with a hydraulic ladder.

A further fifteen minutes went by and still no Fire Brigade, so we just stood in the cold, shivering, discussing various topics including each of ours' Christmas plans, occasionally glancing up at the suspended body. Due to the height the corpse was off the ground and how dark it was, we couldn't quite gauge the approximate age of him. All we could see was that the hanging, lifeless body was a male wearing jeans, training shoes and a zipped-up Parker jacket.

The Fire Brigade eventually rolled up but, to our disappointment, they were in a standard fire appliance only, not the type with an extendable hydraulic ladder. Mike and I confusedly frowned at each other.

'How do they expect us to get him down?' the copper asked, directing his eyes towards the fire crew that were alighting the bright red appliance. The Fire Officer walked towards us as we stood huddled together like three gossiping old women.

'Where's the hydraulic ladder, we can't get him down with one of your normal ladders?' the copper asked him.

'Eh?' he replied.

'How do you suggest we get him down?' I asked.

'I don't know. We weren't told what height he was at or exact position,' he said.

I can't remember to this day why the Fire Officer couldn't request the hydraulic ladder appliance, but he couldn't, and he didn't! Perhaps it was attending to a huge fire somewhere else on Christmas Eve morning. Not likely! So for the next twenty minutes, the copper, Fire Officer, Mike and I discussed various options, all of which had problems; they were either too dangerous, impractical, or we didn't have the appropriate equipment.

By now our night vision had adapted further, and with a gradual increase in daylight, the body was becoming more defined, his face a combination of pale and purple where rigor mortis and blood pooling was evidently setting in. His arms were just hanging down by the side of his body, his legs swinging slowly back and forth. It certainly wasn't a scene for anyone squeamish to experience, I tell you.

Time was ticking but we'd still not come to a safe and sound decision as to how we were going to recover the grim corpse. Then, further police began to arrive on scene, including an Inspector, outnumbering the fire crew. After a rather long-winded discussion with his subordinates and the Fire Officer, the Police Inspector came up with a great idea. This was to find the owner of the factory which was close by, and ask him to come and open up the premises, then to get someone with a fork-lift truck licence to lift someone up to the body on a fork-lift truck carrying several wooden pallets. It seemed to me like an excellent idea, but who was going to volunteer to go up twenty feet and recover the grim corpse that was hanging directly above double spiked railings? I assumed the Fire Brigade; after all, that's right up their street, rescuing people from heights – although this wasn't going to be a rescue, only a recovery.

So the discussion of who would be the best person to be lifted began. The Fire Officer explained to the Police Inspector that although the appliance was in possession of safety harnesses, he would not allow any of his men to be lifted up twenty feet over spiked railings. I'm sure we all thought... why? Whoever did it would be wearing a harness, they weren't going to fall and become impaled on the railings, were they! The Inspector asked what we were all thinking, but the Fire Officer blatantly refused to authorise any of his crew to go up. This debating went on for quite a while, with no compromise whatsoever between the Police Inspector and the Fire Officer; he was adamant none of his fire crew were going to be lifted up on the fork-lift truck.

With all discussions now exhausted and still no compromise or volunteer, and the clock ticking away, Mike stepped forward.

'Sod it, I'll do it then! I'm not arsed about the railings! I'll put the harness on and go up so we can get the hell out of here. It's bloody freezing and I'm knackered.'

Now, although I wasn't Mike's boss, I was technically senior to him, as a paramedic, and ultimately responsible for his clinical actions while attending to a patient, and for his safety during an incident. However, I had no reservations whatsoever about him going up to recover the body. As far as I was concerned, with a safety harness on and a fork-lift truck loaded with pallets, driven by a licensed fork-lift driver, I was confident he would be fine. I wouldn't have authorised him to do so if I'd thought it was too dangerous.

The decision was made and by now the factory manager had arrived, accompanied by a licensed fork-lift truck driver. So Mike put some protective gloves on and was fitted into the harness by a fireman. The fork-lift truck was driven from the factory, with pallets in place, to the bridge, just below the hanging corpse. It was becoming increasingly lighter, and the atmosphere evermore eerie with a clearer view of the body. Mike climbed on to the pallets and crouched down, while the driver slowly lifted his forks upwards towards the figure. Meanwhile, I went and placed an open body bag on to the stretcher, ready for when the corpse was lowered to the ground on the pallets.

Mike had been elevated up towards the body and shouted out to the driver as the forks reached a suitable height for him to be able to reach the body and cut the freight strap. He leant forward and wrapped one arm around the waist, to pull the deceased man closer to his body, so that when he cut the strap the body wouldn't just drop to the pallets; or worst case scenario, fall off the pallets and plummet twenty feet to the concrete tarmac. Imagine what the coroner would have to say if that had happened!

Mike held the body with one hand and pulled his tuffcut scissors from the leg pocket of his trousers with his other hand, and cut the strap, taking the full weight of the dead man in one arm, and then carefully allowed the body to slowly slide through his arm on to the pallet. The driver then lowered the forks gradually and safely to the ground. I assisted Mike from the pallets and commended him for volunteering to go up.

With the body recovered, the grim discovery was now gruesomely clear. The dead man's eyes were partially open and bulging out of his eye sockets, caused by the pressure of the noose around his neck upon the sudden halt from the bridge jump, and also because of the weight of his hanging body pulling down on the noose for quite a while. His mouth was ajar and his tongue was sticking out in a childlike manner. His skin was moribund, pale and purple, and he had a huge non-haemorrhaging gash under his chin, where the HGV hook attached to the strap had lacerated upon his abrupt halt after he'd jumped to his death. His jeans showed evidence of effusions of urine and faeces as the sphincter muscles became deprived of oxygen and thus relaxed post-death. To say that it was a sickening and horrendous experience to witness would be an understatement.

Whatever reasons he had for jumping to his death, we were not likely to find out any time soon, if at all. The copper and I donned some protective gloves and lifted the rigid, cold corpse into the body bag I had placed on to the stretcher. Mike and I then carefully rifled through the man's jeans and Parker coat pockets, looking for anything to identify him by, such as a wallet with driving licence or credit card, but he had nothing in his possession. We zipped up the bag and informed ambulance control that we would soon be conveying the body to the hospital mortuary, which was about eight miles away.

It was by now approaching 8 a.m. and we'd been on scene for nearly two hours. We were just about to start mobilising to the mortuary when, to our surprise, a day crew from the same ambulance station arrived on scene; they were as fresh as a daisy. They hadn't morbidly come to see a man hanging, oh no. The ambulance control room dispatcher, knowing full well we'd had a very busy night of frivolities, verbal abuse and no rest, and were to be back to endure it all again that night, had sent them to change ambulances with us. So they conveyed the deceased to the hospital mortuary instead, and Mike and I headed back to the station to finish the Christmas night shift from hell and go home to our awaiting beds.

Later that day, following a well-earned and much needed sleep, I searched the teletext pages (don't take the piss – I still relied on teletext several years ago) to see if there was any information about the hanging incident, and to my surprise there was, but very little. The only information reported was that a body had been discovered hanging from the Memorial Bridge, and it was that of a twenty-nine year-old male.

However, several days later, the incident appeared in the local rag and the deceased twenty-nine year-old was identified by name. He had recently split with his partner, who wouldn't allow him to see his children. I imagine it was a lot more complex than that, but nevertheless enough to send him over the edge, literally! Whatever his reasons were, he must have thought there was no point in him living, because in the early hours of Christmas Eve, while millions of people around the UK were having festive fun, he walked along the bridge footpath, tied an HGV freight strap to the bridge railing, then tied the strap, with its hook connector attached, around his neck and jumped to a very undignified death.

Since attending to that particular hanging, I have experienced several more, some of which resuscitation was attempted but to no avail. All of them young men who felt, for reasons of their own, that life was no longer worth living.

Chapter 8
Something's Not Right!

There are, at times, particular incidents a paramedic attends to where there is almost nothing they can do for a patient, other than get them on board the ambulance and put their foot down; not because they don't possess the skills to manage the patient, but because the patient is far too agitated for them to intervene. For example: head injuries.

When someone sustains a significant head injury from, for instance, falling from a significant height, then often, usually within minutes, the internal bleeding inside the closed box – that is, the skull – can cause pressure to build up, and thus cause the patient to become cerebrally irritated or combative. This causes them, through no fault of their own, to involuntarily thrash about and often hurl obscenities at the ambulance crew or anyone else around them trying to help.

It has to be said that when you witness this, it is quite disturbing, because the prognosis is poor. Unless the pressure is released – by those amazing neurosurgeons who drill into the skull – the pressure increases and pushes the brain down through the small opening at the base of the skull; a term called 'coning'. Once coning occurs, the patient is likely to die… or remain on a ventilator, keeping the patient alive until the decision is made by the family to switch the machine off. In the rare event the patient regains consciousness, they are likely to be severely brain damaged and live – if you can call it that – in a vegetative state for the rest of their life.

This next incident is not related to a head injury but it is about me not being able to assess, diagnose or treat my patient because of how incredibly agitated, uncooperative and incompliant she was. The story begins one lovely spring evening. It was 6:32 p.m. My crewmate, Vic, a paramedic, and I were just thirty minutes from finishing a twelve hour day shift. The day had been very busy, so we were both keen to call it a day. While sat in the station mess room with other personnel, chatting, my hand portable radio sounded.

'Receiving, over,' I said.

'Roger, RED call to Bishop's Fashion Store on Raymead retail estate to a sixty-six year-old female complaining of shortness of breath, over,' the dispatcher said.

'Roger, understood,' I confirmed.

Without delay, we mobilised from the station to the given location and arrived on the retail estate within eight minutes. As we crawled along the access road in the ambulance, looking for the correct store, we spotted a member of staff waving at us to gain our attention. On arriving at the entrance, Vic parked up and we both exited the vehicle. I quickly grabbed the paramedic bag from the saloon of the ambulance and followed the member of staff, who hastily escorted us to the patient. As we approached the patient, I could see her seated on a makeshift chair, shouting out, evidently in absolute agony.

'What the hell's going on here?' I thought. When Vic and I arrived at her side, we were greeted by several other members of staff who were attempting to calm and reassure the rather large lady, who was not only in obvious pain and discomfort, but also appeared to be hyperventilating. 'Hello. My name's Andy, this is Vic, what's the concern here?' I calmly asked a member of the store staff while I crouched down beside the patient, who was breathing shallow and rapidly.

'Well, she was stood at the counter and all of a sudden started panicking and struggling for breath, so we sat her down and called you,' a female member of staff informed me.

'OK... what's your name, my love?' I asked the lady while taking hold of her hand to reassure her.

'J-Je-Jean,' she replied with a fear induced stutter. She appeared extremely flushed, cherry red in fact, in the face, neck and upper part of her chest, which was exposed due to quite a baggy V-neck blouse that she was wearing. The scene was attracting quite a lot of attention from onlookers, so within a minute of arriving, I asked Vic to go and get the carry chair, in order to save Jean from any embarrassment she may have been feeling.

'Right Jean, I'm gonna pop an oxygen mask on you, OK my love? Try and calm down for me though, OK. You're hyperventilating. Now, you have pain in your chest, is that right?'

'It hurts! It hurts!' she shouted, with a panic-stricken tone and fearful expression.

'OK Jean, I understand. Take nice deep breaths for me, and calm down, OK, calm down,' I said, while applying the oxygen mask to her face and switching the oxygen cylinder to high flow.

Strictly speaking, when a person is hyperventilating, therapeutic oxygen in addition to atmospheric oxygen isn't normally required, as oxygen levels are usually adequate. However, I administered oxygen as I wasn't sure whether there was more to Jean's rapid breathing rate than simply anxiety alone. As mentioned in a previous chapter, there are a myriad of serious underlying medical reasons why someone would hyperventilate.

'Now, do you have any pins and needles down your arm, or anywhere else?'

'My chest hurts! It feels tight! Oh God!' she answered while nodding her head at me, gasping for breath.

'OK, calm down, come on, calm down. Now what about pins and

needles down your arm?'

'My left arm! My chest hurts! Oh God!' she shouted, evidently confused, nodding her head, gazing in to my eyes with sheer terror.

'Do you feel nauseas, or have you vomited at all today?'

'N-n-no, it hurts, my chest hurts!'

'OK my love, try and calm down for me, OK.'

While waiting for Vic to return with the carry chair, a man approached me,

'I'm her son,' he informed me. 'Is everything OK?'

'Well, she's in a bit of a state at the moment, so we're gonna get y'mum straight on the ambulance, out of public gaze, chief, OK?'

'Yeah, thank you.'

'Does she regularly have anxiety attacks?' I asked with relevance.

'No. I've never known her to have an anxiety attack, ever!' he answered, shaking his head. That basic bit of information raised my concerns a little, simply because it would be unusual for a sixty-six year-old female to suddenly begin having panic attacks. I was therefore very keen to get Jean on board the ambulance and out of public view, so I could thoroughly assess her, reduce her pain, and also try and diagnose the problem; or at least find anything physiologically or medically untoward going on inside her body.

Vic returned with the carry chair, so I encouraged and assisted Jean to stand and move herself on to it. With Jean still shouting out loudly, complaining of excruciating pain in her chest, and hyperventilating, Vic wheeled Jean out to the ambulance.

Bystanders were gawping as Jean's screaming drew unwanted attention. I asked her son to accompany us while we undertook some tests in the back of the ambulance.

Once we had Jean on board, I calmly asked her to sit in an upright position on the stretcher, as sitting upright might assist her to breathe more controllably, thus calming her down so I could undertake some pertinent tests. But when she moved herself from the carry chair onto the stretcher, she slid herself down and rolled on to her left side, facing away from us. Her feet hung over the end of the stretcher and she continued to breathe at a rapid rate, and scream out loudly in sheer agony.

'Jean, I need you to face forward, hun, so I can do some tests on you. Can you sit up and face forward for me, please?'

'I can't, it hurts! It hurts! My chest hurts! Oh God!' she cried out while rolling about, agitated, on the stretcher.

'I understand Jean, but if you try and keep still and let me do some tests on you, I can take the pain away, OK.'

'Arrrgh... It hurts! I can't breathe! My chest hurts!' she exclaimed once again.

'Mum, calm down and let these guys help you!' Jean's son assertively asked her, as if becoming wound up by her unusual behaviour.

'I can't, it hurts, arrrgh! Please help me, the pain... oh God!'

Jean continued to move around the stretcher, screaming in pain, for a further five minutes, regardless of all of our attempts at trying to calm her down. Her son was becoming increasingly agitated and impatient, and I could feel myself becoming more and more flushed with what was becoming a bit of a nightmare scenario. It was also a safety issue, as we couldn't risk mobilising to hospital if she wouldn't keep reasonably still on the stretcher, for fear of her rolling on to the floor, causing injury and potentially worsening the prognosis. I took a deep breath in through the nose and out through the mouth, slowly.

'OK... Jean, please try and calm down and let us help you. I can take the pain away, trust me, but you need to keep still and let me do some tests first.'

'I can't, it hurts so much... my chest, I can't breathe... it's hurting, please help me!'

'Jean, I can help you but you need to calm down and keep still,' I said, doing my utmost best to remain calm. She continued to roll around. I didn't know what else to do to reassure her. I let out a deep sigh. 'Jean, please try and calm down, I need to check your blood pressure and then I can give you something for the pain, but I will need to put a needle in your arm first. I can't put a needle in your arm while you're rolling around,' I explained with an empathetic tone.

Jean didn't comprehend what I had said to her, she just continued to writhe around the stretcher, agitated, lethargic and in agonising pain, for which I had no diagnostic cause. Vic and I felt nothing short of helpless, as we could do very little to help.

'I tell y'what, Vic, get a blood glucose reading, will y'mate. That's one test we can do while she's rolling around,' I asked, while becoming conscious of myself getting more flushed, agitated and increasingly sweaty from all the commotion.

'She is diabetic. She's a type two. She takes tablets for it, and she's got high blood pressure, too,' Jean's son informed me, while Vic restrained her hand with implied consent and pin-pricked her finger for a drop of blood. Moments later, Vic said,

'Her glucose level is raised, mate; fourteen point five.'

'When did she last eat, chief?' I asked, directing my eyes at her son while Jean continued to scream and roll around anxiously on the stretcher, simultaneously clutching at the mask, trying to pull it from her face.

'About twelve o'clock, I think.'

'Has she taken her medication today?'

'Yeah, I think so.'

'Her blood sugars are a little high, but I don't think this is necessarily a diabetic related problem… more of a consequence of something else occurring… possibly cardiac in nature,' I said, thinking out aloud.

Jean was not presenting with the typical signs and symptoms of a textbook heart attack – by that I mean, part of her heart tissue becoming starved of oxygen, consequently causing heart tissue death. This is often due to a coronary artery occluded by fatty plaque which, if left untreated, will either dissolve by itself, which is rare, or more commonly kill.

Chest pain is a cardinal sign and symptom of a heart attack, but Jean was presenting like no one I'd ever experienced before, especially if she was having a heart attack. In fact, she was probably the most unlikely heart attack presentation I had ever dealt with throughout my entire career to that point – if it *was* a heart attack, that is. I wasn't convinced.

What did go through my mind was the fact that Jean was diabetic. You may have read earlier that it is common for diabetics to suffer a heart attack either with or without pain, and in some instances to feel chest pain without one or more of the other textbook signs and symptoms of a heart attack – for example, pale, sweaty and clammy skin; nausea or vomiting; double incontinence; and fear of impending doom, to name but a few. Jean wasn't pale, sweaty or clammy, she was cherry red. She hadn't complained of nausea and had not vomited. I pondered to myself,

'Could it be that fear of impending doom was the cause of Jean' behaviour?'

'Mum, come on, let them help you, he'll give you summot for the pain if you calm down. Sit up for them, will ya!' Jean's son said once again with assertion.

I couldn't calm or reassure her, so I was unable to safely administer any pain relief or undertake any assessments. We'e been parked up outside the retail store for ten minutes by now and only managed to obtain a measure of Jean's blood glucose. Vi and I could have normally carried out a number of assessments and provided intravenous pain relief in that time. I had no choice but to risk conveying Jean to hospital with her rolling around and no strapped in on the stretcher. However, I was terribly suspiciou that something sinister was occurring. I wanted doctors to see her immediately upon our arrival. I therefore contacted the A&E department direct by mobile telephone to explain the situation to them, prior to us mobilising to hospital. The conversation with a charge nurse went something like this:

'Hello, A 'n' E majors.'

'Hiya, it's Andy Thompson, paramedic. I've gotta bit of a problem. I've got a sixty-six year-old female on board the ambulance. She appears to be hyperventilating, complaining o tightness in the chest and pins and needles down the arm. But she': just rollin' around the stretcher in absolute agony. Can you hear 'e down the phone? I can't get any vitals on 'er. Ideally, I wanna d an ECG and give 'er some pain relief etcetera, but she won't kee still. Can you have resus waitin' for me, with an ETA of eigh minutes?'

'I dunno Andy, we've got your lot queuing up in the corridor, and resus is full at the moment. Sorry mate.' By *your lot* he was referring to other ambulance crews.

'I appreciate that, mate, but I think there's something 'appening with her, but 'cause I can't get any vitals, I can't treat 'er appropriately, or give 'er any analgesia. I think she needs t'be in resus though, mate, I really do.'

'I 'aven't got the room though, Andy, it's chaotic in 'ere, mate.'

'OK but she's gonna be noisy on the ward. I'll keep tryin' to calm 'er on route to hospital, but expect us soon.'

'OK mate, see ya soon.'

I wasn't happy being told there was no room in resus, although being refused a resus cubicle is very rare. I understood to some degree, because the charge nurse couldn't physically see what my concerns were with Jean; he probably assumed that my patient was merely experiencing a non-life-threatening anxiety episode, which seldom requires resus or immediate attention from a doctor, particularly when the A&E ward is chaotic.

We had no choice but to convey Jean to hospital without any pertinent assessments or pain relief administered, as she would not calm down or cease rolling around on the stretcher. Vic began mobilising steadily on blue lights to the A&E department, while I, accompanied by Jean's son, continued with my attempts to calm her as she rolled around shouting,

'My chest! I can't breathe! It's hurting! Please help me!'

'Jean, try and calm down for me please... come on Jean, let me help you.'

'Mum, let 'im 'elp you, he'll give you summot for the pain if you calm down. Sit up for them, will ya!' Jean's son requested yet again.

Jean did not calm and was uncooperative and incompliant during the journey to hospital. At one point she nearly rolled off the stretcher on to the floor, even with the cot-side up; both her son and I leapt forward and stopped her, just in the nick of time.

While on route to hospital, I noticed Jean's partially exposed upper chest progressively changing from the cherry red colour it had been on our arrival and while stationary in the back of the ambulance outside the store, to a more mottled, purple appearance. This observation caused me to become *very* concerned indeed, and I had no observations to assist me with a diagnosis or differential diagnoses. Therefore, I contacted the A&E department again, and the conversation went something like this:

'Hello, A 'n' E majors.'

'Hi mate, it's Andy again. Sorry but I really need resus for my patient, she's gettin' worse, she's screaming out in agony. I want a doctor to see her straight away. She's still agitated and won't let me do anything for her, but there's something going on. I 'aven't got a clue what, but something's not right mate, I'm tellin' ya, something's not right. Her chest is goin' mottled.' He let out a big sigh.

'OK. I'll clear a resus cubicle for ya.'

'Cheers mate, I appreciate that. ETA now five minutes, OK?'

'OK, see ya in a bit.'

I hung up and shouted to Vic, through the small window situated between the cab and the saloon of the ambulance, that I'd contacted A&E and that the doctors would be awaiting our arrival. I also informed him that Jean was deteriorating and had become mottled in appearance, and would he therefore drive with a little more urgency, regardless of the fact that Jean was continuing to throw herself around the stretcher, still in unbearable pain.

Throughout the remainder of the short journey, Jean's chest became more and more mottled; and the mottling began spreading to her face and arms. She was becoming a living corpse right in front of my eyes. And I felt absolutely helpless. I couldn't even get her to leave the oxygen mask over her face. Every time I adjusted it back in to position, she simply pulled it back off, probably feeling suffocated by it as anxious patients often do.

When we arrived at the A&E department, Vic vacated his seat and hastily opened the rear doors. We quickly wheeled the stretcher into the resus room, where a doctor and a nurse were awaiting our arrival. Jean continued to clearly emphasise the amount of pain she was in. The two medical staff awaiting our arrival took one look at how much pain she was in, and how mottled her face, chest and arms were, and looked directly at me with their eyes wide open, as if in utter shock at her disturbing presentation.

We quickly transferred her onto the hospital bed, but due to Jean's agitation and the noise she was making, I was unable to offer the medical team any handover; there was far too much commotion to even consider it. Instead, I explained to the staff that Jean had not kept still throughout my entire time with her, because of the pain in her chest; hence I had no observations, with the exception of a blood glucose reading which I reported was a little high but nothing to be concerned about. Also that her chest had gone from a cherry red colour to a purple, mottled appearance over a few minutes.

Even while on the hospital bed – which is a lot more comfortable than an ambulance stretcher – Jean continued to thrash around in agony.

'Arrrgh! Please help me, it hurts!'

'Jean, calm down please, calm down, I can help you, but please calm down,' the senior doctor asked without success. Jean tirelessly shouted out as if in the most unimaginable pain. The doctors and nurses tried to calm her and ascertain a history of events, but with no joy. I was stood next to the nurse, trying to help them calm Jean so they could start assessing what was wrong with her. The nurse turned to me,

'Andy, can you try and get a blood pressure for us, mate?' she asked.

'Yeah, I've had no luck though in the ambulance; she's been like this throughout.' So I wrapped the cuff of the automatic blood pressure monitor around Jean's left arm, with great difficulty due to her moving around the resus bed. After a struggle, I finally managed to secure the cuff in place, so I pressed the start button. The cuff inflated as normal and then began to deflate, which was also normal. However, it fully deflated and wouldn't display a blood pressure reading. That usually meant that either the patient's blood pressure was too low for the monitor to be able to make an accurate measurement, or the movement was causing the machine to fail. I removed the cuff from her arm and wrapped it around the calf of her left leg instead, again with great difficulty.

Meanwhile, the nurse had managed to position the ECG leads, one on each of Jean's four limbs and also six leads across her left breast. That was done in order to analyse the rhythm of the heart from twelve different angles, which would identify whether Jean's anxiety and pain in her chest had anything to do with her heart.

My attempts at measuring a blood pressure on Jean's calf proved successful; the monitor displayed a reading of 75/45mmHg, which was life-threateningly low. The doctors managed to calm Jean a little, which was fortunate because ECG recordings do not print legibly with excessive movement, even with a built-in filter to minimise disturbance. The nurse pressed the record button on the ECG monitor and the ECG began analysing the rhythm of Jean's heart. Several seconds later, the machine automatically printed a recording. I immediately handed the printout to the doctor; he had a quick look at it and then handed it back to me, so I had a quick look, too. What it displayed surprised me: it suggested that Jean may have been having a heart attack. The most unlikely patient presentation of a heart attack I had ever seen.

The significance of the ECG recording suggested that the occlusion was potentially in a coronary artery that supplied the rear side of her heart, which was less common and would therefore require blood tests and a further, more appropriate and alternative type of ECG analysis to confirm a diagnosis and treat accordingly.

The doctor and nurse did their utmost best to secure intravenous access, in order to administer analgesia to Jean. However, that proved unsuccessful too, due to her moving about, and because she was quite a large lady. Large people are often quite difficult to cannulate, as the excess fat on the arms 'hides' the veins, as it were. An anaesthetist was therefore called to the cubicle with a view to attempting cannulation, sedating and intubating her, so that blood tests, further ECGs, x-rays and other pertinent observations could be undertaken.

I wasn't party to the further assessments and treatment of Jean as I went into another room to complete my paperwork, while Vic replaced the linen on the ambulance stretcher, and also tidied up the vehicle's saloon a little, ready to hand over to the night crew. By the time we were ready to clear from the hospital, Jean's agitation had improved very little. Her condition had yet to be fully diagnosed and confirmed, as an anaesthetist had still not arrived fifteen minutes after their attendance had been requested. Vic and I left the A&E staff to continue their attempts at assessing and treating Jean, and informed ambulance control that we were clear from the hospital and were returning to the station to book off-duty.

On the way back to the station, Vic and I discussed the incident.

Neither of us had ever seen a patient behave so agitated whil
having a heart attack; not even a patient with a severe head injur
usually presents as agitated as she had. I had never experienced
patient in such anguish and torturous pain before I attended t
Jean, nor have I ever since, to the day I am writing this story. I
was quite a disturbing situation to experience, I have to admit.

A couple of days later, while handing over a patient to an A&I
sister, I spotted the nurse who had been involved in the assessmer
and treatment of Jean, so I approached her and asked what ha
happened after we'd left. She informed me that Jean deteriorate
further and eventually went in to cardiac arrest, about twent
minutes or so after Vic and I had cleared from the hospital, an
although advanced life support measures were attempted
defibrillation, CPR, intubation and ventilation, drug and flui
therapy – she was sadly pronounced dead at about 7:45 p.m., les
than an hour and a half after Vic and I received the treble-nine cal
to attend to her experiencing a *panic attack* in the retail store.

The nurse also told me that the doctors not only had a high inde
of suspicion that Jean was having a heart attack, but also that the
suspected another, underlying cause of her death, which wa
unable to be diagnosed before Jean sadly passed away.

Chapter 9
As Thick as Thieves

I don't want to sound naïve, but you would think that health care professionals – including paramedics – would be able to go about their daily working lives without having to take their own personal safety into account when tending to a patient. And when I say personal safety, I mean without being verbally or physically attacked by the patient or a patient's friend or loved one. Why on earth would anyone want to attack a doctor, nurse or a member of an ambulance crew, verbally or physically? They're the very people who are there to help. However, assault on NHS staff is common and is on the increase.

Posters are displayed in the saloon of ambulances and around hospital wards to warn a patient or anyone accompanying a patient, that acts of aggression or abuse will not be tolerated, and if anyone does abuse or assault NHS staff, then they will be prosecuted. I can't speak for other health care professions, but when it happens to ambulance personnel it isn't always reported, neither to the police, nor to their line manager. The excuse for not doing so is usually down to not having the time to complete the paperwork involved, as ambulance crews get very little downtime.

My biggest pet-hate in life is bullies and those that intimidate people, particularly if the bully is bigger than his chosen victim, which is usually the case. I myself have experienced, on three separate occasions, acts of aggressive behaviour from patients who were of the bullying and intimidating ilk; two of which I will not go in to exact detail here of how I managed those situations. Did I report them? No. I didn't have the time; too much paperwork! Besides, justice was done, as far as I was concerned!

The other occasion, which I will detail here, happened during a road traffic collision I attended. While I was dealing with a motorcyclist who had life-threatening injuries, I received aggressive and threatening verbal abuse from his uninjured pillion passenger.

The story begins one gorgeous, hot summer's day. It was 4:30 p.m. and it had been a very busy and tiring shift thus far of which Simon, a reasonably experienced technician, and I only had two and a half hours left to complete. We were awaiting the arrival of a community midwife, as we had just assisted a mum in the delivery of her second baby. The delivery had gone very smooth, with the exception of the umbilical cord being wrapped around the baby's neck. However, that was common and easy to deal with, so there was no need for concern.

At approximately 4:45 p.m. the midwife arrived, and after liaising with her for ten minutes or so, she decided that the traumatised but elated mother did not need to go to hospital. Therefore, Simon and I congratulated the mother for the umpteenth time and then vacated the address from the front door, towards our parked ambulance. As I closed the garden gate behind us, a middle-aged gentleman was getting out of his car, close by. He informed us that there had been a crash at the crossroads between Grants Road and the Expressway slip road, about two minutes' drive away. So Simon and I hastily placed our equipment back into the vehicle and I informed ambulance control that we were clear from the address... and to no surprise, we were immediately passed information regarding the incident that had occurred on the crossroads a short distance away.

The call was given to us as a motorcyclist versus car, and that the motorcyclist was carrying a pillion passenger. We were also informed that we would be the first crew on scene and that further crews would be dispatched when available, but to give them a 'sit-rep' (situation report) on our arrival at scene. We mobilised towards the scene with blue lights and sirens in operation for the short journey, anticipating that another 'proper job' – delivering a baby is a 'proper job' too – was looming.

When we arrived at the location, Simon parked the ambulance in a 'fend off' position, so a motorist didn't plough in to us while rubber-necking. Not that you would think anyone could miss a bright yellow ambulance, the size of a motorhome, parked up in the road with lights flashing and plough in to it, would you? Think again, I have known that to happen. I vacated the cab and grabbed the equipment from the saloon of the ambulance, including the gas and air as I could clearly hear someone shouting out as if in agony, using almost every expletive in the English language.

I began walking the twenty yards towards a crowd of seven or eight people who were stood, gathered around a male lying flat on his back on the tarmac, all in a commotion; not actually attempting to provide first-aid, just all in a commotion. There was evidence of severe blood loss, which had soaked through his jeans from his right leg on to the road. Even from twenty yards away, I could see his leg was facing southwest as opposed to south, so it was blatantly obvious he had sustained a serious fracture; and from the amount of blood evident, quite possibly an arterial bleed from the same leg, too.

There was another young male stood near to the motorcyclist, who I assumed was the pillion passenger. He didn't appear to have any obvious injuries but seemed very anxious and was pacing about. And there was also a lady in her late twenties and a teenaged female stood by their car, which was dented on the driver's side door. They both looked uninjured but clearly shaken and upset.

I stopped midway from the crowd and contacted ambulance control via my hand portable radio.

'Ambulance control, go ahead, over,' the dispatcher said.

'Roger, sit-rep. I've got four patients, one seriously injured. Three others stood, appear uninjured but require assessment. I'm requesting two further ambulances and police attendance, over.'

'Roger, understood.'

I then continued towards the crowd. As I arrived within a few feet of the motorcyclist lying flat on the floor, I was immediately met with aggressive verbal abuse from the man I rightly assumed was his pillion passenger.

'Urry up will ya, y'fuckin' prickkk, do summot or he's gonna fuckin' die la!' the skin-headed man said, with an evidently plastic scouse accent. A sudden surge of adrenaline began to circulate my body.

'OK, chill out dude, there's no need to swear at me. I'll see to him, OK,' I calmly stated, while using my free hand to emphasise a calming gesture.

'Get 'im in the fuckin' ambulance and take 'im to fuckin' 'ospital then!'

The shocked crowd witnessing his aggression looked on but offered no assistance, and although the patient's presentation needed my immediate attention, I daren't begin assessing him until I was sure the brain-shy low-life a few feet away wasn't going to attack me.

'Look pal, I will get 'im in the ambulance, but I'm not just gonna move him before I've assessed him, OK. Now, just calm down.'

'Fuck assessin' 'im, just get 'im to 'ospital la or I'll fuckin' twat'ya!'

'Hey! Let me do my job! Move away from him now and give me some space, will ya!' I shouted to him, as a further surge of 'fight or flight' adrenaline shot through my veins at his aggressive and threatening comment. Like I said, my biggest pet-hate in life is those of the bullying and intimidating ilk.

'Do y'job then and get him to fuckin' 'ospital la!' he repeated once again, splaying his arms in an aggressive manner.

'You speaking to me like that is gonna delay me treating him. Now back off! And move away from him, now!' I instructed, with aggression in my tone.

I was infuriated. I understood that people panic under conditions like this, where a friend or loved one is in danger, but there was something about his manner that gave me the impression that he wasn't panicking because of his friend, who was losing a lot of blood from his leg, but panicking for some other reason that I couldn't quite put my finger on.

I felt like educating him of the fact that, as a paramedic in the modern day ambulance service, I can and am expected to do a lot more than just simply put a patient into the back of the ambulance and convey them to hospital, with no assessment or treatment whatsoever; with the exception of a cerebrally irritated or uncooperative patient, that is. However, I refrained, as I suspected he was too thick and ignorant to understand such an explanation. Pillion, as I'll call him, promptly did as I requested and moved several metres away from me. I asked the onlooking crowd to move away from the injured motorcyclist too, to give us space to go to work.

Simon knelt down next to the motorcyclist who continued to scream out in pain, which was a good sign that he had a patent airway and was breathing adequately. On the other hand, he was in so much pain that I don't think he had acknowledged the exchange between me and his pillion. Simon immediately took hold of the seriously injured motorcyclist's head and neck to provide manual in-line immobilisation to his c-spine. Meanwhile, I began questioning him,

'What's y'name, mate?' I asked.

'Arrrgh... fuck! Kevin,' he cried out.

'OK Kevin. How old are y'mate?'

'Twenty-six,' he informed me with a grimacing expression.

'Right Kevin, I need you to keep very still for me. Simon's got hold of y'head and neck as a precaution because you've been thrown from your motorcycle. Now I need to assess you, before we get you onto the ambulance, OK?'

'Arrrgh... fuck! Yeah man!'

'Do you have pain anywhere other than your right leg at all, like neck or back pain?'

'Fuck, no man... just my fuckin' leg!'

Regardless of his answer, I had to take into account that the pain he was experiencing in his leg was potentially distracting pain from anywhere else; for instance, in his neck or back. I looked down at his injured leg. As I had first thought, he had evidently sustained an 'open' mid-shaft femur fracture – 'open' meaning the bone was protruding through the torn leg of his jeans – and blood was pouring out. However, I needed to straighten the injured leg before applying a box splint. That was going to be the tricky bit, because straightening his leg would be extremely painful.

His injuries were obviously life-threatening and therefore time-critical, so I had to assess and treat him fast! Firstly, I needed to minimise the bleeding before I straightened the leg or provided any pain relief, as it was bleeding profusely, causing him to appear pale, sweaty and clammy to the touch. He needed oxygen, so applied the sats probe to his index finger and, while I waited for the figures to appear on the digital display, prepared the gas and air, which takes seconds to do. Moments later, the sats monitor displayed a figure of ninety-seven percent, which was adequate.

'OK Kevin, I'm gonna need to straighten y'leg out, OK? It's gonna hurt but I can give you gas 'n' air for now, to ease the pain, while I prepare something stronger. But I'll need to put a needle in your arm to give you summot stronger, OK?'

'Fuck yeah man, just give me summot!'

I instructed Kevin how to self-administer the gas and air; that meant he was getting supplemental oxygen and analgesia simultaneously. I palpated for a pulse in his wrist, to gauge an approximate systolic blood pressure measurement. He had a palpable pulse pounding at a rate of 125 bpm. The pain may have contributed towards the fast heart rate, but I had to assume it was due to blood loss.

While he was getting high on laughing gas, I opened some large ambulance dressings and carefully applied them tight around the gaping wound of his right leg, regardless of the fact that they may be disturbed when I cut up the leg of his jeans and straighten the leg out. I had no choice, the bleeding needed controlling, and quickly!

With the bleeding now under some degree of control with direct pressure applied, I cut the sleeve of his jacket and positioned a tourniquet to his right arm, removed a large bore cannula from its packaging, and waited several seconds for the veins of his arm to swell with blood. Kevin was experiencing some relief from inhaling the gas and air, but he was still very agitated and still in severe pain. Extending and restraining his right arm, I carefully pierced the skin with the sharp needle, entered the vein and advanced the needle further; a flashback appeared. I unclipped the tourniquet and gradually withdrew the needle fully, disposing of it in the sharps container, leaving the clear plastic tube in his vein. I then screwed the Luer-Lock to the end of the cannula, flushed it with sodium chloride and secured it in place with an adhesive dressing.

I hastily set up a bag of fluid, which I attached to the cannula via the giving set, and beckoned a bystander over to hold the bag of fluid up for me. I then opened the clamp slightly, so the contents were administered to Kevin at a very slow rate.

The next part of my rapid treatment plan was to prepare an anti-sickness drug and morphine. As I was preparing the drugs, I questioned a bystander about how the crash had occurred.

'What 'appended 'ere, mate, d'ya know? Did y'see it?'

'Yeah, he went through a red light at the crossroads at about thirty, thirty-five and T-boned that car,' he said, pointing toward the dented vehicle that the two young females were stood by, still evidently shaken and upset. 'He hit the car door and went 'ed-first over the roof and landed where he is now, an' obviously his mate fell off as well,' he informed me.

What frequently happens when a motorcycle hits a moving or stationary object – for example, T-boning a car – is the motorcycle stops suddenly, projecting the rider forward head first. As the rider is thrown forward from a seated position on the motorcycle, a thigh, or sometimes both thighs, strikes the handlebars with such force that it fractures a femur, or sometimes both femurs. As mentioned in an earlier chapter, femur fractures, whether 'open' or 'closed', are time-critical, as death can occur from exsanguination (bleeding to death) if major arteries are ruptured and if the site of the ruptured artery is not quickly located and 'clamped'.

'Were they both wearing helmets?' I asked, to ascertain the possibility of Kevin having sustained a head injury.

'Yeah, both of 'em, but they both took 'em off before you arrived.'

'OK, cheers mate, thanks for your help.'

Ideally, I would have preferred the helmet to have been left in place and then carefully removed by myself and Simon in a specific way taught during training, in order to minimise further c-spine damage in the event that c-spine damage had occurred.

Now I had the information I needed, and the IV drugs prepared, I progressed with my treatment of Kevin by administering the anti-sickness drug to him, to allow it to start working prior to me giving him the morphine. Although Kevin had a palpable radial pulse, an accurate blood pressure measurement was of paramount importance, so that was the next part of my plan before administering any opiate based analgesia – the morphine, that is. I wrapped the cuff of the blood pressure monitor around the upper aspect of his right arm, inflated it and placed my stethoscope midway up his arm, where the brachial pulse is. After several seconds of deflating the cuff and listening for the appropriate sounds, I obtained a systolic blood pressure measurement of 95mmHg.

Having that accurate measurement meant I could administer IV analgesia and meticulously continue to administer fluid to maintain a palpable radial pulse. The last thing I wanted to do was increase Kevin's blood pressure too much with fluid, as that would mean a higher pressure forcing blood out of his injured, haemorrhaging leg, thus causing an even greater blood loss.

'How's the pain at the moment, Kevin, with the gas 'n' air?' I asked.

'Fuckin' shit… it's killin', man.'

'OK, I'm gonna give you some morphine now. We'll let that take effect and then I'll 'ave to move y'leg, OK?'

'Arrrgh… yeah, whatever man. Just fuckin' do it.'

With the bystander still very helpfully holding the bag of fluid up, I shut the clamp off, to avoid any of the morphine entering the bag, while I slowly administered two point five milligrams of morphine into the cannula. I then re-opened the clamp very slightly.

As I waited to see what effect the morphine had on Kevin's pain and blood pressure, and while Simon continued to immobilise Kevin's c-spine, I pulled my tuffcut scissors from my trouser leg pocket and began slowly cutting off his sock and training shoe, and up the left-hand side trouser leg. His left leg didn't appear to be showing signs of deformity, nor was Kevin complaining of any pain in his left leg. I palpated for a distal pulse in his foot. Moments later, a pulse was palpable, so I wrote an 'X' on the point with my pen.

A couple of minutes had gone by and the morphine was having some, but little effect. Kevin had become slightly less agitated and vocal, but still periodically hurled obscenities. I was trying to work at speed and I could feel the effects of adrenaline hurtling through my body, because I was still pissed with the pillion's aggressive approach and threats towards me. I felt again for a pulse in Kevin's wrist; he still had one. It was beating at 130 bpm.

I undertook a further blood pressure reading to gauge whether the fluid was having the desired effect following the administration of morphine. His post-morphine blood pressure measured 90mmHg, but Kevin was still evidently in pain. So I clamped the fluid again, administered a further two point five milligrams of morphine, and then re-opened the clamp a little further than before – this allowed the contents to drip through the cannula at a faster rate, to counter the blood pressure-reducing effects of morphine that often occur when haemorrhaging is present.

After a couple of minutes, allowing the second dose of morphine to take effect and reduce his pain further, it was time to attempt to straighten his right leg out. It was still going to be painful, but I had to crack on and get him to definitive care ASAP.

'OK Kevin, on a scale of zero to ten, how would you score your pain?'

'It's killin', man,' he replied.

'I understand, Kevin, but I'm gonna 'ave to move it. So how would'ya score it now?'

'Arrrgh, fuck… about a seven, man.'

'OK. Just grit y'teeth and keep sucking back on the gas 'n' air, OK.' I began carefully straightening his leg out in small, gradual movements, but the pain for Kevin was still intense.

'Arrrgh, fuck… fuck!' he screamed out, as I began slowly realigning the leg.

'OK Kev, inhale on the gas 'n' air, mate, while I move y'leg.'

'Arrrgh, fuck y'bastard!'

'Sorry Kev, just keep on the gas, mate.'

'Arrrgh… Fuckin'ell!'

After several periods of moving the leg a little at a time, the intense pain being managed with gas and air, morphine and plentiful obscenities, his leg was eventually facing south again. Kevin continued to self-administer the gas and air. Meanwhile, I began cutting off his right sock and training shoe, and up the right leg of his jeans with my tuffcut scissors, carefully skirting around the already applied dressings. As I was cutting and got closer to his thigh, the full extent of his injuries became apparent. The handlebars of his motorcycle had practically severed his leg off. Almost the entire upper thigh was wide open and I could visibly see the muscle tissue – bubbly yellow fat tissue – flesh and his femur bone protruding. It was an absolute mess and still evidently bleeding.

'How the hell they are going to fix this, I don't know,' I thought 'He's gonna lose this limb, surely?'

The entire limb was exposed and onlookers began moving further away in disgust, with their hands held over their mouths. One or two began retching at the sight of the almost severed limb. I began removing rolled up bandages from their plastic packaging and carefully stacked them, like building blocks, around the protruding bone, before applying a compression bandage around and over the top. Additional compression bandages were placed over the one I'd earlier applied, with further bandages around the rest of the open thigh wound to minimise bleeding and infection.

With the leg straightened and Kevin a little more relaxed, carefully applied a box splint to his fractured leg, with the assistance of a bystander, and then ran to the ambulance to fetch the stretcher and all of the immobilisation equipment, which included the scoop stretcher, rigid c-spine collar, head-blocks and straps.

When I returned to Kevin's side, I attempted to apply a rigid c spine immobilising collar to his neck while Simon continued to provide in-line manual c-spine immobilisation, but Kevin would not tolerate it. They're not meant to be comfortable, but some patients just cannot keep one on. Attempting to keep a rigid c spine collar in place, when the patient cannot tolerate it, generally causes more movement in the patient and a greater risk of worsening c-spine damage than if they are not wearing one. So it occurred to me that although the mechanism of Kevin's injuries warranted full immobilisation, he wasn't going to tolerate any of it and it would be best if we just positioned him onto the scoop stretcher, and refrain from using any immobilisation equipment.

As Simon was crouched holding Kevin's head, I could see, in my peripheral vision, that Pillion was approaching again, against the advice of the gawping bystanders who were trying to calm him. I'd remained calm on the outside all this time, even though my heart had been beating rapidly throughout from trying to work fast while dealing with Pillion and Kevin's time-critical, life-threatening injury.

'Here we go again,' I thought. At the same time, I could hear sirens approaching from the distance and assumed it was the police or one of the two ambulance crews I'd requested. Pillion got closer, arms splayed and an 'I'm 'ard' bounce in his step. That really irritates me, that – the barrels under the arms bounce.

'Are y'gonna get 'im in the fuckin' ambulance or what likkke?' My adrenal glands provided a little more fight or flight juice.

'I've told you, let me do my job. I've got an ambulance on its way to have a look at you too, so chill and wait for it, OK?'

'I don't need a fuckin' ambulance, I'm coming wit' you la.'

'I'll decide that, not you! And no, you're not!' I said, ready to pounce if he came close enough for me to feel remotely threatened, or he showed any signs of an intention to attack me.

'Why the fuck not la?'

'Because I said so… now move away, now!' Meanwhile, the noise from the sirens got closer and closer, and then the tones of the sirens stopped; it was the traffic police arriving. Pillion hurriedly walked away. 'That's odd,' I thought, 'either my comment worked or he's keen to leave now the cops have arrived.'

One of the two coppers approached me, and the other one walked towards Pillion. The copper, observing how badly injured Kevin was, helped me and Simon to carefully place each half of the scoop underneath him, before I clipped the two halves together. We then lifted Kevin the twenty yards to the ambulance, up the ramp and into the saloon, and placed the scoop onto the stretcher.

While in the back of the ambulance, the copper asked me if it would be appropriate for him to ask Kevin a few questions relating to the accident, and undertake an alcohol breath test there and then. I quietly informed him that Kevin had sustained potentially life-threatening injuries and it would therefore not be appropriate for him to undertake a breath test at that time, and that he would probably not get an opportunity at the hospital for some considerable time either, due to the extent of his injuries. The copper stepped out of the ambulance and so we continued our assessment and treatment of Kevin.

Simon undertook a further blood pressure, pulse rate and blood glucose, attached Kevin to the ECG monitor, and assessed his pupillary response, which was normal. Kevin's systolic blood pressure was measuring 90mmHg. The ECG monitor displayed that Kevin's heart rate was regular but now pounding at 125 bpm; he was still compensating and would need immediate attention from the doctors upon our arrival at hospital.

By now the second dose of morphine was having further effect on Kevin's pain, as he gradually became less agitated on the stretcher, but still too irritable to secure him with head-blocks and straps. However, his reduced movement did give us the opportunity to cut his upper garments off, so he was almost entirely exposed; although I covered him with a blanket for dignity purposes, regardless of the scorching heat. Kevin's leg had been straightened and box splinted; he was on the scoop; I'd got the vital observations that I needed; and I'd gained IV access and administered analgesia and fluid. So we were ready to mobilise to A&E.

'Right Simon, I'll contact A'n'E and tell 'em I wanna trauma team on standby. You get us in on blues, mate,' I instructed him, with a sense of urgency in my tone.

The two ambulance crews I'd requested had arrived and had been on scene for a couple of minutes. We were just about to mobilise to A&E when one of the crew opened the side door of the ambulance and informed me that he was taking the pillion passenger through to hospital for a precautionary check-up.

'What! He's finally calmed down?!' I thought. I warned him that the pillion didn't possess a brain and so to be careful, as he'd become aggressive with me several minutes earlier, before their arrival. He also explained that the other attending crew were taking the teenaged passenger of the colliding car through, too, also for a precautionary check-up. The driver of the car was assessed at the scene and did not need hospital treatment, but would travel to hospital with the teen.

I had put the pre-alert message in to A&E, and Simon had begun mobilising to the hospital with blue lights and sirens. With Kevin now less agitated but still not stable, I continued to question his perceived pain score on route, periodically administering further morphine while frequently monitoring his blood pressure; it brought his pain score down to a three out of ten.

Kevin had ceased inhaling on the gas and air, so I placed an oxygen mask over his face and administered oxygen to him. His blood pressure did drop on route to hospital, so I had to set up a second bag of fluid and administer further sodium chloride to him, in order to keep it at an adequate level.

On arriving at the hospital ambulance bay at 5:30 p.m., Simon opened the rear doors and we promptly wheeled the stretcher down the ambulance ramp and into the resuscitation cubicle. The trauma team was gloved and gowned and ready to receive Kevin. Within seconds of arriving in the cubicle, the team lifted the scoop from our stretcher and onto the resus bed. I then gave my handover to the lead doctor, which went something like this:

'This is Kevin, motorcyclist, twenty-six years old. At approximately 1650 hours, he collided with a car and went over the roof at approximately thirty to thirty-five mile per hour, with a pillion passenger on the bike. Helmet worn, but removed by himself prior to our arrival.

'On arrival at scene, AVPU – A. GCS fifteen. Kevin has got a severe, right-sided, open mid-shaft femur fracture. Box splinted after leg straightened following analgesia. Unable to confirm palpable pedal pulse. Left leg assessed; no pain complained of, no deformity, and pedal pulse marked with an 'X'.

'There was evidence of severe blood loss at scene. Mechanism of injury cannot rule out pelvic or spinal injury. No evidence of significant head injury.

'On examination, sats were ninety-seven percent. Gas and air initially self-administered prior to morphine. Blood glucose normal. His ECG rate has been approximately one hundred and twenty-five per minute throughout. Regular monitoring of his blood pressure on route has fluctuated, but remained around ninety systolic with IV morphine and a one litre fluid challenge through large bore IV access in the right arm.

'Kevin was initially very agitated with the pain until analgesia administered. His current pain score is three out of ten after a total of ten milligrams of morphine. He's also had ten milligram of metoclopramide.

'Full c-spine immobilisation warranted but would not be tolerated by Kevin. Gas 'n' air ceased so O-two administered on route. Are there any questions?'

'No. Thank you,' the lead doctor replied.

The medical team then continued with Kevin's assessment and treatment, which Simon and I weren't party to because we went outside to complete the paperwork and tidy up the back of the ambulance a little. As we were doing that, a police officer from the scene of the crash approached us. He informed us that while we were on route to hospital, it had been confirmed that Kevin and Pillion had stolen the motorcycle and helmets from an address on an estate nearby the scene of the crash, just minutes before running a red light and colliding with the car.

'Aha! So that's why Pillion was as aggressive and panicky as he was,' I thought. 'And why he hurriedly walked away from me when the cops arrived.'

Had Kevin been riding the motorcycle faster, he may well have killed himself, his pillion, and quite possibly the two young occupants of the car, too.

Kevin was stabilised in the A&E resus department. His x-rays showed no evidence of spinal injury, but he had fractured his pelvis. He underwent extensive surgery on his injuries and was later transferred to the Intensive Care Unit (ICU).

Pillion came off unscathed and was discharged from A&E shortly after arriving. Fortunately, the teenaged occupant of the car Kevin had collided with was also discharged from hospital uninjured, a short time after arriving at A&E. Kevin's leg was saved by those wonderful surgeons and he was subsequently discharged from hospital.

Less than twelve months later, according to the press, Kevin and Pillion pleaded guilty in court to the theft of a motorcycle and dangerous driving. However, despite possessing previous criminal records, for their thoughtless actions – putting the lives of others at risk, theft of a motorcycle, dangerous driving, and not possessing a brain – they both only received a community service order.

The British Criminal Justice System, don't you just love it?!

The Dark Side

Chapter 10
Sweet Dreams

It was 7 a.m. on a beautiful, sunny summer's morning and I was stuck in work for the next twelve hours, not knowing what the day would bring. I was working with Colin, an experienced paramedic. It would be wrong of me to say he'd seen it all, because that's impossible, but I think it is fair to say he'd seen most things over a career spanning nearly four decades. I think he joined the Ambulance Service before electronic audible warning devices were invented, and the 'siren' was the ambulance driver's crewmate ringing a bell out of the window.

During the early days of his career, the PTS and the emergency ambulance service were combined. Therefore, an ambulance man – I say ambulance man and not paramedic because paramedics didn't exist in the ambulance service four decades ago – would pick up the old dears and, while conveying them to their out-patient appointments, would attend to emergencies. So, for example, they might be called to a fatal car crash and put the deceased onto the stretcher alongside the other patients, drop off the patients at their appointments and then go immediately to the mortuary. I'm not joking, it really did happen! Can you imagine that being accepted practice today? I can see the headlines now: *'Ambulance Takes OAP to Hospital with Decapitated Body Lying on Stretcher Shock Horror!'* There would be outrage.

Anyway, the first five hours of the shift were unusually quiet – that's the Q word in the ambulance service. You mustn't use the word 'quiet' irresponsibly. That is frowned upon because it can have serious consequences; the general public start to pick up their telephones and inadvertently dial 999 with no control or thought whatsoever.

At noon on this particular quiet day, while Colin and I were still sat in the station mess room relaxing, a member of the public picked up their telephone and dialled treble-nine. Not because a member of staff had irresponsibly used the word 'quiet', but because something had happened that would change their life, and the lives of others, forever! The station's RED call radio alarm sounded, so Colin shot out of the armchair and pressed the push-to-talk button.

'Station, over.'

'Roger, RED call to a four month old cardiac arrest,' the voice said over the radio, calmly but with an obvious adrenal-fuelled tremor in her voice.

'Shit! Did she just say four month old cardiac arrest, then?' Colin asked me. I didn't answer him because I momentarily froze the second the dispatcher had said *cardiac arrest*, after I'd clearly heard *four month old*. My adrenaline began circulating my body at breakneck speed, and I wasn't even out of my chair yet.

Paediatric emergencies are every ambulance personnel's worst nightmare. No one wants to attend to a severely sick or injured child – no one. But, like I stated earlier, it goes with the territory. And I wouldn't have joined the ambulance service if I'd have thought for one second that, in the event I did attend to a severely sick or injured child, I wouldn't cope. I knew that during my career there was a strong possibility that I would see dead children, and I accepted that.

So Colin and I threw our cups down and sprinted down the stairs, out of the station door and into the ambulance. With blue lights and sirens wailing, I swiftly drove to the estate, doing my utmost best not to allow red mist to get the better of me and affect my driving skill. The address given to us was on an estate notorious for being difficult to find door numbers because of the architectural layout. However, I knew exactly where I was going, and exactly where the address was!

I rolled up to the concrete jungle-like estate, braking hard and almost forgetting to apply the handbrake because of the sheer haste of wanting to get to the patient.

'What was the door number again?' Colin asked, shaking with anticipatory adrenaline.

'It's that one there,' I said, pointing directly at a white uPVC door. We exited the ambulance, swiftly grabbed the appropriate equipment from the saloon and power walked towards the marginally open door. Colin was a little in front of me. As we approached the garden pathway, we heard a female screaming hysterically. My own breathing rate suddenly increased with the anticipation of what I was about to endure.

As we stepped over the threshold and into the house, we were met by a young teenaged father pacing up and down the lounge in a panicked state and crying while holding a baby, with just a nappy on, in one arm and a cordless telephone in the other hand. He was being given CPR instructions by the ambulance control room call-taker, but unfortunately had no hands free to perform the actions given to him. The young teenaged mother was understandably too hysterical to assist her partner.

'They're here, they're here!' he informed the call-taker, with a grief-stricken tone and simultaneously crying in absolute despair. Colin practically snatched the baby from his arms. It appeared lifeless, his whole face and body was grey. Tinges of purple stained his skin. His tiny little eyelids were closed, covering his eyes. He appeared to be in a peaceful, deep sleep.

Colin hurriedly walked towards a dining table, with me following closely behind. He placed the infant on to its back and quickly checked inside his mouth for mucous, vomit or a foreign body that may have been obstructing his airway – the possible cause of the cardiac arrest – but the airway was clear. He then pulled the infant BVM from the kit bag, attached it to the oxygen cylinder and quickly ventilated the infant with five squeezes of the bag, before compressing the chest of his little body with two firm fingers.

Simultaneously, I began applying the ECG leads, one to each of his four tiny limbs, with bucket loads of adrenaline causing my hands to shake while trying to peel the sticky, gel-covered electrodes from the plastic. With ECG leads in place, I switched the monitor on and sadly, but no surprise to me and Colin judging by the colour of the little fella, it displayed a 'flatline'.

From the start of my ambulance service career, up until that particular day, I'd never seen what a dead child looked like, let alone a four month old baby. I don't know why I ever thought that in the unfortunate event I ever did see a dead baby, it would look any different to a dead adult, which I'd seen plenty of, but it did. And I knew from the appearance of him that the outcome was not going to be a positive one: he was grey, cold and rigor mortis had already begun setting in. Unbeknown to his parents, he had been dead for quite a while and no amount of CPR was going to bring him back to life. However, Colin and I commenced CPR.

While medically futile, by me and Colin being seen to begin CPR it would help the parents to grieve in the long term following the impending loss of their four month old infant. By watching us resuscitate their beautiful baby, they would hopefully remember, for the rest of their lives, that we had tried, and that alone can help the grieving process when someone loses a loved one, particularly a child.

If we'd had the slightest notion that he could have been revived, when we arrived at the address, we would have immediately taken him from his dad's arms and carried him straight to the ambulance, accompanied by one or both of his parents. I would have put my foot down all the way to A&E, with Colin doing CPR in the back throughout the entire journey, as opposed to attempting resuscitation in the house – that only delays the time it would have taken to get him to further professional care from an abundance of doctors.

In some UK districts, it is protocol to convey a child to hospital performing CPR regardless of their presentation when an ambulance crew arrives at their side, with the exception of decapitation or other obvious traumatic injuries that are not compatible with life. However, in my honest and professional opinion, I think it is ethically and morally wrong! If a health care professional honestly believes that a child has been deceased for some considerable time, based on rigor mortis and a 'flatline' ECG rhythm, then what good does it do for the parents whisking their child off and acting as if you believe, as a paramedic, that everything is going to be OK if the baby is rushed to hospital? It does nothing but cause the parents further distress, and offers mentally damaging false hope.

Close by in the background, while we were performing basic life support, all we could hear was angst, panic, crying and the parents' footsteps pacing back and forth on the laminated floor, eagerly awaiting for us to turn to them and say, 'everything's going to be alright.' Colin and I both had our heads down throughout, not wanting to look at each other's facial expressions because we knew what the outcome was going to be.

'Right Andy, I'll keep doing ventilations, you take over the compressions.'

'OK mate,' I sombrely replied.

So, there we were, Colin ventilating and me pushing down on the baby's chest at a rate of one hundred times a minute; regardless of the fact that the baby was presenting grey in colour, rigor mortised and the ECG displayed a 'flatline'. Although we knew what the outcome was going to be, we still continued CPR for a further seven minutes, with no change in the rhythm of the baby's heart. To continue for longer, or to convey him to hospital, would have been all the more distressing for the parents.

The most ethical decision to make was to cease resuscitation whil
the baby was still in the family home, where the parents ha
experienced four joyous months with their little boy, and allo
them to spend a little while longer with him in the same plac
where their memories were created. And that's what we did.

We both agreed, by way of facial expression and a subtle nod, t
cease resuscitation. Colin placed the BVM down and I stoppe
compressions but left the monitor switched on, displaying
'flatline', as I was going to have to print a sixty-second stri
identifying what the exact rhythm was – and the exact time whe
death was pronounced – for the purpose of the police and th
coroner.

Colin took it upon himself to break the news to the young teenag
couple that their baby was dead; a conversation I wasn't party t
because Colin had asked me to go to the ambulance and discreetl
inform the control room call-taker that the baby was dead o
arrival and that resuscitation, although undertaken, had in fact bee
futile. I also had to request the police, who would alert SOCC
(Scenes of Crime Officers) because a baby had suddenly died, a
home; they would have to rule out foul play. I had no concern
whatsoever that foul play was the cause of his death, but then
was no forensic expert.

I went back into the house and Colin had broken the news to th
young couple, and as you can imagine, they were absolutel
devastated, to say the least. I can't even begin to imagine what i
must be like to lose a child of any age, but they only had fou
months with him. They couldn't comprehend what had happened
and neither could I.

It sounds harsh, but to cry or show too much emotion whil
dealing with the death of a patient would be perceived a
extremely unprofessional in the emergency services, even when
baby has died. You're expected to remain strong and resilient fo
the parents, even under such sad and tragic circumstances. It's O

to be sympathetic or even console a family member or relative who has just lost a loved one in your presence, but cry – no, that is forbidden. You are expected to keep it together until you get back to the ambulance station.

Colin carefully picked up the baby from the table, cradled it in his arms and told both of the parents to sit down on the sofa together. They both huddled in close, and then he passed their lifeless only child into his mum's arms.

'There you are, you hold him, give him a cuddle, talk to him, tell him how much you love him,' he said in a soft and sympathetic tone. The young mum held him in her arms, stared at his face and stroked his cheek,

'Sweet dreams, little man,' she said, sobbing her heart out.

I heard sirens approaching our location, so I went outside to see who it was. An RRV paramedic pulled up with his blue lights flashing. He had been given the same call as us and sent as backup, but he had responded from quite a distance away. By the time he had arrived, we had already ceased resuscitation attempts. When he saw me stood outside, he slowed his pace down from a sprint to an amble, knowing full well from my facial expression that resuscitation had been ceased. After a quick conversation regarding the circumstances, he promptly cleared with ambulance control and responded to a further treble-nine call.

I went back inside, where the young couple was spending those extra precious moments with their baby. They sat on the sofa cradling him, stroking him and repeatedly kissing his forehead. Watching them was one of the hardest, most gut-wrenching experiences I've ever had in my entire life, let alone my career.

Colin began tactfully and carefully questioning the parents as to what had happened prior to calling treble-nine. Still sobbing but having temporarily calmed down a little, they explained to Colin that Charlie, the deceased, had recently been suffering with a cough and cold and had been frequently disturbing throughout the night, but they had been regularly monitoring him. When they awoke, having slept-in due to a disturbed night, they found him unresponsive in his cot, so the father ran downstairs with him in his arms and dialled treble-nine.

Colin began documenting the baby's full name, date of birth and the circumstances surrounding Charlie's death, on to the patient report form and ROLE form, which needed to be thorough as he, or both of us, would likely have to go to coroner's court in the distant future. When the police arrived, accompanied by SOCO, I felt really uncomfortable. This teenaged couple's baby was dead but the police have to, by law, 'snoop' around the house and ask the youngsters some very awkward questions in order to rule out suspicious circumstances; although, I have to say, they approached the situation with exceptional tact. Colin liaised with the police and handed over a copy of the 'flatline' ECG rhythm strip and the documentation he had completed, and then we vacated the premises.

We both took a deep breath, climbed back into the cab of the ambulance, and then I drove the ambulance away from the address with as little engine noise as possible, out of respect, and then headed back towards the ambulance station. It was going to be a very sombre day for Charlie's parents, as they were going to have to begin the grieving process, co-operate with the police, and have Charlie taken from their loving, clutching arms so he could be conveyed to the mortuary. And if that wasn't enough, they were going to have to break the devastating news to their family and friends. It doesn't bear thinking about, does it.

Historically, when ambulance personnel attend to the death of a child or other distressing incident, they are understandably offered some downtime back at the ambulance station, to reflect, discuss and even to cry and express their emotions if they so wish. The ambulance service does have counsellors in place for events like the one we had dealt with. However, although some members of staff do utilise said counselling, the majority of staff find counsel in either the crewmate they were working with at the time of the traumatising, sad or tragic incident, or with another member of ambulance staff, and sometimes with their own loved ones.

While Colin and I were parked up at A&E discussing the incident, he looked at me with an inquisitive frown.

'Andy, I've been thinking all afternoon how did he know which exact house to drive to on that estate? The estate is a logistical nightmare. How did you know?'

'I used to be a postman, remember? I used to deliver mail to that estate, so I know exactly how the houses are numbered... as sad as that may sound. I'd give a cabbie a run for his money though, I tell ya,' I humorously replied, with a half-hearted grin.

'Oh yeah, I forgot you used to be a postman, that explains things,' Colin said, smiling back at me.

The light humour was our way of coping, I suppose.

Later that evening at around 6:50 p.m., ten minutes before Colin and I were due to finish our shift, the red telephone rang, which is used by ambulance control to pass emergencies as an alternative to the station's RED call radio alarm. Colin answered it, and with a scrap piece of paper and a pen to hand, he started scribbling the address and details of the emergency. I simultaneously looked over Colin's shoulder as he was writing. He put the phone down.

'I'll go and pass this to the night crew; they should be ready to go out by now.'

'Hang on, Col! That's the address we were at this afternoon... Charlie, the baby,' I said with concern as to why they needed an ambulance to the same address we attended just seven hours ago.

He inquisitively looked down at the scrap piece of paper in his hand.

'Oh yeah, you're right! The job is to an elderly female collapsed but conscious. I'll go an' 'ave a quick word with the crew an' explain to them what 'appened this afternoon.'

Colin and I could only assume that the elderly female 'collapsed but conscious' was Charlie's great grandma, and was understandably finding it difficult to come to terms with the events that had occurred that day.

Several months later, I was reading the local rag and came across the coroner's inquest into the cause of Charlie's death. It was confirmed that Charlie died of Sudden Infant Death Syndrome (SIDS), more commonly known as 'cot death'. Surprisingly, though fortunate, neither Colin nor I had been summoned to coroner's court.

Sadly, each time I drove passed the house where Charlie had lived with his young parents, I had a momentary flashback to the day I saw his little lifeless body and his distraught parents, and wonder whatever happened to them. Did they have another baby? Did the ordeal split them up, as the loss of a child regularly does? I don't know, and it's probably best that I never know.

Since attending to the death of Charlie, and unbeknown to me at the time, over the following eighteen months I would assist in the delivery of two unexpected stillbirths, and also attend to a two month old baby who had also died from SIDS. And while sat writing this true story about the most unimaginable, sad and tragic loss anyone could possibly endure, with a little reminiscent tear in my eye, I can't help but think that sometimes life can be so cruel.

Epilogue

Well, that's it. Of course, there are more memories I could share with you, some in great detail and others... well, I only have brief memories of. For example, the man found on Halloween morning face down in the shallow water of a certain canal, with a crow bar embedded in his back. It turned out he was a paedophile from Manchester. One man and two women were later charged with his murder.

Then there's the young man who stormed out of his house following a row with his fiancée, only to drive so erratic that he crashed through a barrier and into a tree, and was killed instantly. How do I know about the row with his fiancée? Because I attended to his mum several weeks later; she had collapsed at home following chemotherapy treatment. There were an excessive number of pictures of him around the lounge, almost like a shrine. She explained to me where and when he had died, and the history of events leading up to the crash. I never mentioned that I was the paramedic that had pronounced her son dead at the scene.

And then there's the young farmer who, one late evening, went out to his barn and shot himself in the chest with a shotgun. It turned out he had cattle related financial worries and had been suffering depression as a consequence.

It's not all grim though, oh no! Being a paramedic often brings humorous incidents too. For example, I was once passed an emergency call and when I arrived on the correct estate given to me by ambulance control, I mistakenly knocked at the wrong address. When the occupant opened the door, looking rather puzzled as to why a paramedic was on his front step, I said,

'You did ring for an ambulance, didn't you?'

'Two years ago, yeah,' he said, with a confused expression on his face.

'Well I apologise for the delay, sir, but we have been exceptionally busy,' I replied.

Then there's the middle-aged bloke who I spent twenty minutes trying to convince couldn't be the father of the baby in his twelve week pregnant, teenage mistress's womb... who he had only met three weeks previous! He wouldn't take my word for it though. He was adamant that the baby was his. I politely informed him he didn't need to be Carol Vorderman to figure that one out. Unbelievable! He wouldn't know which way an elevator went if you gave him two guesses.

Then there's the bloke who tried to convince me he was ex-SAS, and should have been involved in the storming of the Iranian Embassy in London but was on leave from 'The Regiment' when the siege took place. However, he hadn't done his history homework and so became somewhat red-faced when I looked at his date of birth – that he had given me while completing my paperwork – and informed him he would have only been seventeen years old when the Iranian Embassy siege took place in 1980. Needless to say, his basic arithmetic wasn't up to scratch, either.

And then there's the one about the sixteen year-old couple who had the house to themselves and decided to 'sexually experiment', with extremely embarrassing, painful and bloody consequences, especially for him. The young lad only went and tore his banj... no, I won't.

Anyway, I hope you've enjoyed reading this book as much as I did writing it, I really do, because maybe, just maybe, I'll begin putting pen to paper again to share a further selection of my experiences with you in considerable detail. If in the meantime, while you have been reading this book, you've been contemplating a career as a paramedic, then I only have one piece of advice for you: be careful what you wish for, because it might just happen!

Layman's Terms

A&E: Accident & Emergency

ABC: Airway, Breathing and Circulation.

Adrenaline: A drug used in cardiac arrest and other medical emergencies to increase blood pressure and cardiac output.

Ambulance Dispatcher: A senior ambulance service control room operator who dispatches the nearest health care professional/s to the location or address of a patient.

Ambulance Technician: A lesser qualified and skilled member of an ambulance crew.

Analgesic: Pain relief.

Aneurism: A swelling or enlargement of a part of an artery, resulting from weakening of the arterial wall.

Asystole: A 'flatline' ECG rhythm – signifying the heart is no longer pumping blood and there is no electrical cardiac activity occurring.

Atropine: A drug used to increase the heart rate.

AVPU Scale: A method of assessing a patient's level of consciousness by determining whether a patient is Alert, responsive to Verbal or Painful stimuli, or Unresponsive. Used principally in the initial assessment.

Benzyl Penicillin: A gold standard form of an antibiotic drug.

Box splint: A rigid or flexible appliance for fixation of displaced or movable parts, usually used to immobilise fractured limbs.

BVM: Bag Valve Mask – used to ventilate patients who are not breathing, or are breathing inadequately.

Cannula: A needle for inserting into a vein to administer drugs and/or fluids.

Cannulation: The skill of inserting a needle into a vein, then withdrawing the needle, leaving a plastic tube in place, to administer drugs and/or fluids.

Cardiac Arrest: An absence of breathing and a pulse.

Carotid Pulse: A pulse point located in the neck. Usually signifies a systolic blood pressure of at least 60mmHg.

Charge Nurse: A male equivalent of a senior female nurse i.e. a Sister.

Claret: Blood.

Cold Response: A response not requiring the use of visual and audible warning devices.

Control Room Call-Taker: A control room operator who ascertains information from a caller when they telephone the ambulance service via a 999 call.

CPR: Cardio-Pulmonary Resuscitation – the process of attempting to resuscitate someone by mechanically emulating the work of the heart and lungs by compressing the chest and blowing air into the lungs.

C-spine: The cervical spine – housed and protected by the first seven vertebrae in the spinal column.

Defibrillator: A machine which delivers a controlled electric pulse across the chest to make the heart restart when it has stopped beating effectively.

Diastolic: The arterial pressure during the relaxing phase of the heart.

Entonox: Gas and air – an analgesic.

Femur: Thigh bone.

GCS: Glasgow Coma Scale/Score – a neurological scale that aims to give a reliable, objective way of recording the conscious state of a person for initial as well as subsequent assessments. A patient is assessed against the criteria of the scale, and the resulting points give a patient a score between 3, indicating deep unconsciousness or an absence of breathing and a pulse, and 15, alert and responsive.

Giving Set: Fluid administration equipment.

Haemorrhaging: Bleeding.

Handover: To verbally convey information about a patient, from one health care professional to another.

Hot Response: A response requiring the use of visual and audible warning devices.

Hyperglycaemia: High blood sugar.

Hypertension: High blood pressure.

Hyperventilating: Rapid, shallow breathing.

Hypoglycaemia: Low blood sugar.

Hypotension: Low blood pressure.

Hypovolaemic Shock: Shock due to insufficient blood volume, either from haemorrhage or other loss of fluid, or from widespread vasodilation so that normal blood volume cannot maintain tissue perfusion.

Hypoxia: Inadequate oxygen in the tissues of the body.

Immobilisation: A process of limiting movement, or making incapable of movement.

Intubation: The skill of placing a tube down a patient's windpipe in order to ventilate them when they're not breathing, or breathing inadequately.

IV Access: Intravenous access.

IV Glucose: A bag of fluid containing 10% glucose, used to treat hypoglycaemic patients.

Laryngoscope: A handle with a rigid, blunt, curved blade equipped with a source of light, used for moving a patient's tongue to the left to view the vocal chords.

Longboard: Rigid, stretcher-like equipment used for immobilising and securing suspected spinal cord injured patients onto.

Meningococcal Septicaemia: A form of blood poisoning caused by a specific bacterium.

Mess Room: A social/refreshment lounge within the ambulance station.

Metoclopramide: An anti-nausea/sickness drug.

Morphine Sulphate: An opiate based analgesic.

Normoglycaemic: Normal blood sugar.

NPA: Nasopharyngeal airway – a small tube inserted into a nostril to provide a patent airway.

Oesophagus: The food pipe in the human body.

'O' Negative Blood: The universal blood group that can be infused into anyone regardless of their specific blood group type.

Out-Station: A station outside of your normal base station.

Paramedic Bag: A bag/rucksack containing the majority of equipment a paramedic will ever need, excluding the bulky equipment.

Pedal Pulse: A pulse point located in the foot.

Plastic Scouser: A person from outside of the City of Liverpool who acquires a strong Liverpudlian accent (scouse) in order to make others believe he/she is a true Liverpudlian.

Pre-alert: A message conveyed to a hospital department prior to the arrival of the patient by ambulance.

PRF: Patient Report Form.

Prophylactic: Preventative.

PTS: Patient Transport Service – the non-emergency aspect of the NHS Ambulance Service.

Pyrexic: A high temperature.

Radial Pulse: A pulse point located in the wrist. Usually signifies a systolic blood pressure of at least 80mmHg.

RED Call: 999 Emergency requiring visual and audible warning devices to be utilised while on route to the location of a patient.

Resus: Resuscitation department – for severely sick or injured patients.

Rigid C-spine Collar: A device used to immobilise a patient's neck or c-spine.

Rigor Mortis: Post death stiffening of the body.

ROLE form: Recognition of Life Extinct form.

RRV: Rapid Response Vehicle – manned by a solo responder, usually a paramedic, but technicians do man them in some ambulance services.

RTC: Road Traffic Collision.

Sats/Sp02: A measure of how oxygenated the blood is.

Scoop: A stretcher that divides in two halves – used for lifting patients from the ground onto an ambulance stretcher.

Scrote: A male with low character, who is idle, thoughtless, inconsiderate, disrespectful, with bad manners, no moral fibre and often with a poor appearance.

SIDS: Sudden Infant Death Syndrome, aka cot death.

Silent MI: A heart attack where the victim does not experience chest pain.

Situation Report: A report giving the situation of an incident, from an attending crew's perspective – also called a SITREP.

SoCO: Scenes of Crime Officers.

Sodium Chloride: 0.9% saline fluid – used to flush cannulas or increase the body's internal fluid volume.

Sphygmomanometer: Equipment for measuring blood pressure.

Stethoscope: An acoustic medical device for listening to interna sounds in a human.

Supine: Lying flat on the back.

Systolic: The arterial pressure during contraction of the heart.

Tourniquet: A constricting device used to allow blood to engorge the veins prior to cannulating.

Trauma Team: A group of doctors and nurses on standby to receive a trauma patient from an ambulance crew.

Triage: A French word meaning 'To Sort'. Patients are triaged to enable an order of priority for assessment and treatment from Health Care Professionals.

Triple 'A': Abdominal Aortic Aneurism.

Tuffcut Scissors: Robust scissors used in emergency medical response and rescue to cut through clothing – for example, leather motorcycle jackets, trousers, boots etc.

12-Lead ECG: Only 10 leads to be precise, but it analyses the rhythm of the heart from 12 different angles. Used to assist a paramedic diagnose various conditions. However, its primary purpose is to diagnose heart attacks.

Urgent Call: A call that has been triaged as non-life-threatening, therefore not requiring visual and audible warning devices.

Ventilating: Assisting a patient to breathe using manual or mechanical means.

Vital Signs (Vitals): The key signs that are used to evaluate the patient's overall condition, including respiratory rate, pulse, blood pressure, level of consciousness, skin characteristics and much more.

Lightning Source UK Ltd.
Milton Keynes UK
UKOW01f0630301017
311869UK00012B/533/P